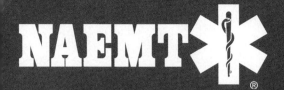

In Cooperation With

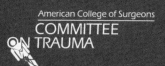
American College of Surgeons
COMMITTEE
ON TRAUMA

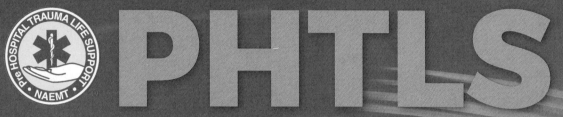

PHTLS
Prehospital Trauma Life Support
NINTH EDITION

Course Manual

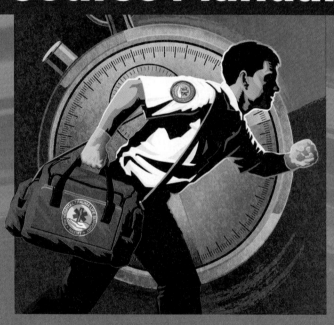

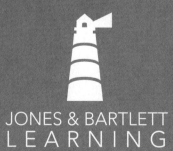

JONES & BARTLETT
LEARNING

Endorsed By

east
Eastern Association for the
Surgery of Trauma

Special Operations
Medical Association

AAOS
American Academy of Orthopaedic Surgeons

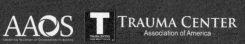
TRAUMA CENTER
Association of America

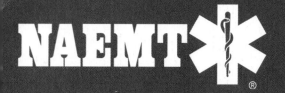

In Cooperation With

American College of Surgeons
COMMITTEE
ON TRAUMA

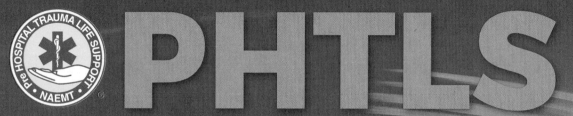

PHTLS

Prehospital Trauma Life Support

NINTH EDITION

Course Manual

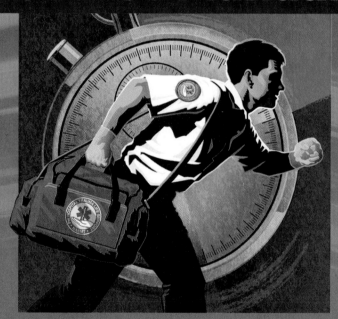

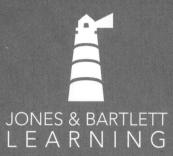

JONES & BARTLETT
LEARNING

Endorsed By

Eastern Association for the
Surgery of Trauma

Special Operations
Medical Association

AAOS

TRAUMA CENTER
Association of America

World Headquarters
Jones & Bartlett Learning
5 Wall Street
Burlington, MA 01803
978-443-5000
info@jblearning.com
www.jblearning.com
www.psglearning.com

Jones & Bartlett Learning books and products are available through most bookstores and online booksellers. To contact the Jones & Bartlett Learning Public Safety Group directly, call 800-832-0034, fax 978-443-8000, or visit our website, www.psglearning.com.

Substantial discounts on bulk quantities of Jones & Bartlett Learning publications are available to corporations, professional associations, and other qualified organizations. For details and specific discount information, contact the special sales department at Jones & Bartlett Learning via the above contact information or send an email to specialsales@jblearning.com.

17144-0

Production Credits

General Manager and Executive Publisher: Kimberly Brophy
VP, Product Development: Christine Emerton
Senior Managing Editor: Donna Gridley
Product Manager: Tiffany Sliter
Product Development Manager: Jennifer Deforge-Kling
VP, Sales, Public Safety Group: Matthew Maniscalco
Director of Production: Jenny L. Corriveau
Project Specialist: Robert Furrier
Director of Marketing Operations: Brian Rooney
Production Services Manager: Colleen Lamy
VP, Manufacturing and Inventory Control: Therese Connell
Composition: S4Carlisle Publishing Services
Cover Design: Kristin E. Parker
Text Design: Kristin E. Parker
Media Development Editor: Troy Liston
Rights & Media Specialist: Thais Miller
Cover Image (Title Page, Part Opener, Chapter Opener):
 © Ralf Hiemisch/Getty Images
Printing and Binding: LSC Communications
Cover Printing: LSC Communications

Library of Congress Cataloging-in-Publication Data

Names: National Association of Emergency Medical Technicians (U.S.), author.
Title: PHTLS : prehospital trauma life support course manual / National
  Association of Emergency Medical Technicians.
Other titles: Prehospital trauma life support
Description: First edition. | Burlington, Massachusetts : Jones & Bartlett
  Learning, [2020] | Includes bibliographical references.
Identifiers: LCCN 2018053934 | ISBN 9781284171457 (pbk.)
Subjects: | MESH: Wounds and Injuries--therapy | Emergency Medical Services |
  First Aid--methods | Wounds and Injuries--diagnosis | Advanced Trauma Life
Support | Case Reports
Classification: LCC RA975.5.E5 | NLM WO 700 | DDC 362.18--dc23
LC record available at https://lccn.loc.gov/2018053934

6048

Printed in the United States of America
23 22 21 20 19   10 9 8 7 6 5 4 3 2 1

Brief Contents

Table of Contents

Preface

The National Association of Emergency Medical Technicians (NAEMT) and the NAEMT Prehospital Trauma (PHT) committee, along with our partners at Jones & Bartlett Learning Public Safety Group, are excited to present the first *Prehospital Trauma Life Support (PHTLS) Course Manual* to accompany the ninth edition of the PHTLS course and textbook.

Revising the PHTLS course was a true labor of love, and the PHTLS course author team took the team approach very seriously when starting this mission. They carefully considered feedback from PHTLS faculty around the world for input on best PHTLS teaching practices. Course lessons now follow a case-based approach that encourages critical thinking and student engagement. These cases are reflected in the course manual.

The *PHTLS Course Manual* was created to enhance the course experience for all participants. The ninth edition PHTLS textbook will continue as the gold-standard reference book, containing the full spectrum of medical science in the area of prehospital trauma care. It is designed for use by students and instructors before, during, and after the course.

This new course manual presents content specific to the course lectures and case studies, and it highlights key knowledge from the course lessons to give you, the student, a deeper understanding of the content. It includes content presented by the instructor so that you can access this information after the course.

The PHT committee designed the ninth edition of the PHTLS course to utilize both the textbook and the course manual to ensure that students receive the maximum educational benefits before, during, and after the 16 hours of classroom content.

Course Editor—Ninth Edition

John C. Phelps II, MA, NRP, ACHE
PHTLS Course Editor, PHT Committee
NAEMT State Education Coordinator, Texas
Assistant Professor, Department of Emergency Health
  Sciences
University of Texas Health San Antonio
San Antonio, Texas

Acknowledgments

© Ralf Hiemisch/Getty Images.

PHTLS Course Author Team

Faizan H. Arshad, MD
EMS Medical Director, Health Quest
   Systems
Lead Author, All Hazards Disaster
   Response
NAEMT PHT Committee, EMS Physician
   Representative
Host and Producer of EMS Nation Podcast
Evaluations Subcommittee Chair,
   Hudson Valley REMAC
Hudson Valley, New York

Amie Fuller, NRP
PHTLS Affiliate Faculty
Lieutenant, Frederick County Fire
   and Rescue
Winchester, Virginia

**Anthony Harbour, BSN, MEd,
   RN, NRP**
Virginia PHTLS State Coordinator
   (1989–2016)
PHTLS Affiliate Faculty
Acute Care/EMS Educator, Center for
   Trauma and Critical Care Education
Virginia Commonwealth University,
   School of Medicine
Director, Southern Virginia EMS
Roanoke, Virginia

Jim McKendry, BSc, MEM
PHTLS Affiliate Faculty
Director, Paramedic Association of
   Manitoba
Instructor, Paramedicine, Red River
   College
Winnipeg, Manitoba, Canada

Jean-Cyrille Pitteloud, MD
At-large Member, PHT Committee
Head of Anesthesiology, HJBE Hospital
Bern County, Switzerland
Chair of the Board for Acute Care
   Anesthesia, the Swiss Society of
   Anesthesiology (SGAR)
Sion, Switzerland

PHTLS Course Manual Editor

Nancy Hoffmann, MSW
Director of Education, Publishing
National Association of Emergency
Medical Technicians

Contributors

PHTLS Course Contributors

James Bayreuther
Sean Britton
Riana Constantinou
Shawn Couch
Jan Fillipo
Cody Jenkins
James Jensen
Lara Marcelo
Joanne Piccininni
Victor Pimentel, MD
Dawn Poetter
Neil Pryde, MD
Lee Richardson
Sarrissa Ryan

Thank You

**Oberfeldarzt Divisionär Andreas
   Stettbacher, MD**
Swiss Army Surgeon General
Federal Department of Defense
Ittigen, Switzerland

Bryan Ware, EMTP
Fire Chief
Beulah Fire Protection District
Beulah, Colorado

Prehospital Trauma (PHT) Committee

**PHTLS–Medical Director
Alexander L. Eastman, MD, MPH,
   FACS, FAEMS**
Medical Director and Chief,
   The Rees-Jones Trauma Center
   at Parkland Memorial Hospital
Division of Burns, Trauma, and
   Critical Care, University of Texas
   Southwestern Medical Center
Lieutenant and Chief Medical Officer,
   Dallas Police Department
Dallas, Texas

Faizan H. Arshad, MD
At-large Member, PHT Committee
EMS Medical Director, Health Quest
   Systems
Lead Author, All Hazards Disaster
   Response
NAEMT PHT Committee, EMS Physician
   Representative
Host and Producer of EMS Nation
   Podcast
Evaluations Subcommittee Chair,
   Hudson Valley REMAC
Hudson Valley, New York

Frank Butler, MD
Military Medical Advisor, PHT
   Committee
CAPT, MC, USN (Retired)
Chairperson, Committee on Tactical
   Combat Casualty Care
Joint Trauma System

Warren Dorlac, MD, FACS
Tactical Medical Director, PHT
   Committee
Col (Retired), USAF, MC, FS
Medical Director, Trauma and Acute
   Care Surgery
Medical Center of the Rockies
University of Colorado Health
Loveland, Colorado

Lawrence Hatfield, MEd, NREMT-P
Technical Advisor, PHT Committee
Lead Analyst, Instructor
National Nuclear Security
   Administration
Emergency Operations Training
   Academy
Albuquerque, New Mexico

John C. Phelps II, MA, NRP, ACHE
PHTLS Course Editor, PHT Committee
NAEMT State Education Coordinator,
   Texas
Assistant Professor, Department of
   Emergency Health Sciences
University of Texas Health San Antonio
San Antonio, Texas

Jean-Cyrille Pitteloud, MD
At-large Member, PHT Committee
Head of Anesthesiology, HJBE Hospital
Bern County, Switzerland
Chair of the Board for Acute Care
   Anesthesia of the Swiss Society of
   Anesthesiology (SGAR)
Sion, Switzerland

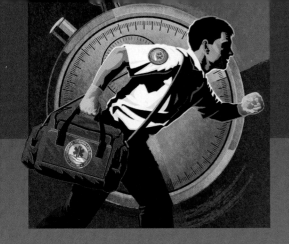

Introduction and Overview of Trauma Care and PHTLS

LESSON OBJECTIVES
- Discuss the societal and financial impacts of trauma.
- Explain the goals, philosophy, and educational approach of Prehospital Trauma Life Support (PHTLS).
- Explain the history and evolution of prehospital trauma care.
- List the three phases of trauma care.
- Discuss the effects of communication and documentation in trauma care.

Introduction

Welcome to Prehospital Trauma Life Support (PHTLS)! This ninth edition of the PHTLS course was created by a team of subject matter experts, including instructors, emergency medical services (EMS) practitioners, and physicians from around the world. They have worked to create a course based on the latest medical evidence and that represents current best practices for prehospital care of the trauma patient.

In this course manual, you will find tips, references, resources, and information to support your learning. It is a companion to the course and a supplement to the PHTLS textbook. As the PHTLS textbook acknowledges, this course ultimately benefits the person who needs our help—the patient. At the end of each run, we should feel that the patient received nothing short of our very best.

Societal Impacts of Trauma

Injuries and deaths from trauma not only have a direct impact on those involved, but on society as a whole. Worldwide, over 5 million people die annually as a result of injury, accounting for 9% of deaths. Motor vehicle collisions (MVCs) and drowning are substantial causes of death in early life. In fact, MVCs and falls are the only causes of death resulting from trauma expected to increase globally by 2030.

The Yin and Yang of MVCs

Examining fall- and MVC-related deaths illustrates some of the complications that are found in addressing unintentional injury and trauma on a universal scale. Although efforts to reduce MVC fatalities have resulted in decreasing numbers of deaths, MVC-related deaths are still expected to increase globally by 2030 because of an increase in the number of vehicles and related infrastructure.

Special Populations: The Rise of Falls

Of fall-related deaths in 2015, 80% occurred in persons 65 years of age and older. There is an increasing number of geriatric patients, and this places a burden on healthcare systems. Previously, there had not been a need to treat such a large population in developing and developed countries. The increase in the geriatric population is mainly due to increased access to basic health interventions.

Examining death rates due to trauma is only the tip of the iceberg. The number one cause of nonfatal injuries in the United States during 2015 was unintentional falls. In fact, unintentional injury is the leading cause of death between the ages of 1 and 45 years. Unintentional injury results in 14,000 deaths each day worldwide. The combined total deaths from diseases such as malaria, tuberculosis, and HIV/AIDS amount to around half as many deaths as those resulting from injury!

CRITICAL-THINKING QUESTION

On an individual level, think of the devastating impact an injury can have on quality of life. Can you think of some examples you have witnessed? Could these injuries have been prevented?

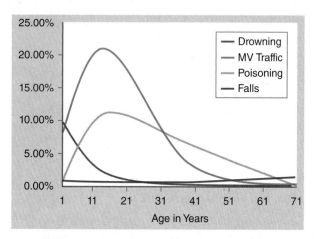

Figure 1-1 Percentage of all deaths by selected cause—ages 1 to 85 years.

Data from the National Center for Injury Prevention and Control: WISQARS. Leading Causes of Death Reports 1981-2015. Centers for Disease Control and Prevention. https://webappa.cdc.gov/sasweb/ncipc/leadcause.html

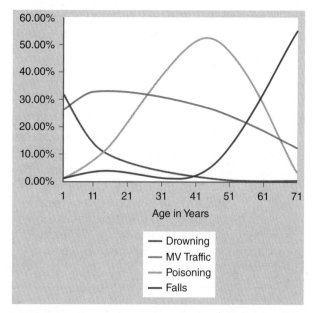

Figure 1-2 Percentage of unintentional injury deaths by selected cause—ages 1 to 85 years.

Data from the National Center for Injury Prevention and Control: WISQARS. Leading Causes of Death Reports 1981-2015. Centers for Disease Control and Prevention. https://webappa.cdc.gov/sasweb/ncipc/leadcause.html

---

FOR MORE INFORMATION

Refer to the "Philosophy of PHTLS" section of Chapter 1: PHTLS: Past, Present, and Future.

Financial Impacts of Trauma

While the loss of life due to trauma is staggering, so too is the financial burden of caring for the victims who survive. Billions of dollars are spent on the management of trauma patients, not including the dollars lost in wages, insurance administration costs, property damage, and employer costs.

The National Safety Council (NSC) estimated a financial impact of approximately $886.4 billion in 2015 from both fatal and nonfatal trauma in the United States. Wages and productivity lost due to trauma was approximately $458 billion annually, more than twice as much as the costs associated with injuries resulting in fatalities. Per patient costs associated with cancer and heart disease are much lower. The NSC's Injury Facts webpage is a great resource to learn more about the societal costs of trauma (https://injuryfacts.nsc.org /all-injuries/costs/societal-costs/).

QUICK TIP

By using the knowledge and skills taught in PHTLS, you can reduce the costs of trauma. For example, protecting a fractured cervical spine properly may make a difference for a patient between quadriplegia and a productive, healthy life with unrestricted activity.

CRITICAL-THINKING QUESTION

What is one change you can make in your daily practice that can help reduce trauma costs in your community?

FOR MORE INFORMATION

Refer to the "Epidemiology and Financial Burden" section of Chapter 1: PHTLS: Past, Present, and Future.

Goals of PHTLS

The goals of PHTLS are simple and clear:

- Reduce mortality and injury from trauma.
- Provide prehospital care providers with knowledge and skills.
- Provide appropriate care to trauma patients.

To help achieve these goals, you will apply your critical-thinking skills in the field. Critical thinking in medicine is a process where the healthcare provider assesses the situation, the patient, and the resources available and uses the information to decide on and provide the best care for the patient. The critical-thinking process requires you to:

- Develop a plan of action.
- Initiate the plan.
- Reassess the plan as care for the patient moves forward.
- Adjust the plan as the patient's condition or circumstances change.

Components of Critical Thinking in Emergency Medical Care

1. Assess the situation.
2. Assess the patient.
3. Assess the available resources.
4. Analyze the possible solutions.
5. Select the best answer to manage the situation and patient.
6. Develop the plan of action.
7. Initiate the plan of action.
8. Reassess the response of the patient to the plan of action.
9. Make any needed adjustments or changes to the plan of action.
10. Continue with steps 8 and 9 until this phase of care is completed.

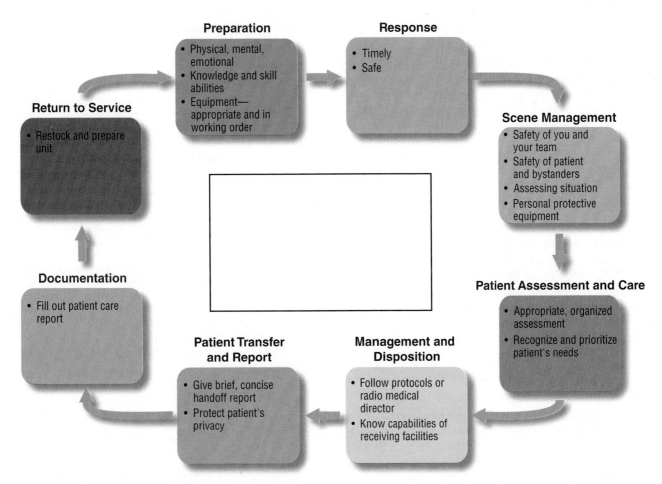

Figure 1-3 Prehospital care providers follow an important sequence of procedures for each emergency call.

© Jones & Bartlett Learning.

FOR MORE INFORMATION

On critical thinking, refer to the "Critical Thinking" section of Chapter 2: Golden Principles, Preferences, and Critical Thinking.

Philosophy of PHTLS

The philosophy of PHTLS hinges on:

- Research
- Interventions
- Patient care delivery

Research—What Do We Know?

In recent years, there has been an increase in research specific to prehospital care. Many of the old, established prehospital standards of care are being challenged by evidence-based research. For example, tourniquets are no longer considered a tool of last resort, and advanced airways are increasingly questioned in the prehospital setting. Another area being widely investigated is the use of backboards and spinal immobilization techniques. Prehospital care is ever-changing, and its best practices are based on applying evidence-based medicine in the best interests of the patient.

Research provides us with the foundation for the best practices in trauma care. It validates or contests current practices and determines future practices. All research must be critically evaluated to determine whether the findings apply to EMS systems and patient populations before a practice can be changed.

QUICK TIP

Throughout the ninth edition of the PHTLS textbook, the evidence from research studies is cited, described, and discussed to help you make the best choices for your patients based on your knowledge, training, skills, and resources.

Prehospital Research Resources— Get Involved!

Suggested journals for prehospital research include but are not limited to:

- *Prehospital Emergency Care*
- *Journal of Trauma*
- *Annals of Emergency Medicine*
- *Journal of the American College of Surgeons*
- *Journal of Emergency Medicine*
- *Academic Emergency Medicine*
- *Emergency Medicine Journal*

Organizations involved in or supporting prehospital research:

- UCLA's Prehospital Care Research Forum
- Fisdap
- National Association of EMS Educators
- National Highway Traffic Safety Administration Office of EMS

Websites to visit include:

- http://prehospitalresearch.eu/
- https://one.nhtsa.gov/people/injury/ems/Archive/EMS03-ResearchAgenda/home.htm
- https://www.cpc.mednet.ucla.edu/pcrf

QUICK TIP

Prehospital care providers should be involved with research in prehospital care.

Interventions—What Do We Do?

Appropriate interventions in prehospital trauma care are based on the assessment of each patient. Often, knowing when *not* to do something is more important than knowing when to do it. Although this course focuses on trauma interventions, PHTLS neither recommends nor prohibits specific actions for the prehospital care provider. Appropriate skills and interventions are determined by local protocols and by critical cost-benefit evaluation.

Patient Care Delivery—How Do We Do It?

Patient care delivery focuses on delivering the trauma patient to the right facility, utilizing the right mode of transport, in the right amount of time, as safely as possible.

FOR MORE INFORMATION

Refer to the "Philosophy of PHTLS" section of Chapter 1: PHTLS: Past, Present, and Future and the "Research" section of Chapter 2: Golden Principles, Preferences, and Critical Thinking.

Team Approach

PHTLS stresses using a team approach for patient care that includes a variety of players ranging in knowledge and skills. The team approach goes beyond just patient care—it also includes research, data collection, and prevention programs that can help decrease the number of traumatic events each year. The players on the trauma prevention, assessment, and care team include:

- Citizens
- Dispatchers
- Law enforcement
- Fire personnel
- Highway safety experts
- Hospital personnel
- Rehabilitation services
- Primary care providers

Trauma is a global problem, and prevention is a vital part of our job. Working together provides trauma patients with the highest chance of survival.

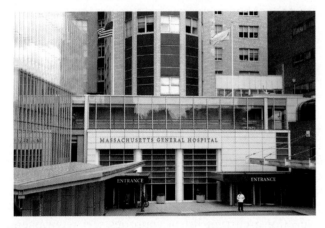

Figure 1-4 Working together—both in the field and in the hospital—provides trauma patients with the highest chance of survival.

© Elise Amendola/AP images.

CRITICAL-THINKING QUESTION

Who is on your local team? Think beyond your colleagues within the service where you work.

A New Approach to the Assessment and Treatment of Trauma Patients

Traditionally, PHTLS provides an understanding of anatomy and physiology, the pathophysiology of trauma,

and the assessment and care of the trauma patient. In the ninth edition of the course, there is a new focus on using the XABCDE approach to patient assessment. Patients who are bleeding or breathing inadequately do not have much time before their condition results in disability or becomes fatal.

XABCDE

The ninth edition of PHTLS, introduces a new approach to the primary survey that recognizes the immediate and potentially irreversible threat posed by exsanguinating extremity or junctional hemorrhage. The "X" placed before the traditional "ABCDE" describes the need to address exsanguinating hemorrhage immediately after establishing scene safety and before addressing airway. Severe exsanguinating hemorrhage, particularly arterial bleeding, has the potential to lead to complete loss of total or near total blood volume in a relatively short period of time. Depending on the pace of the bleeding, that time can be just a few minutes. Thus, even prior to airway stabilization, controlling severe bleeding from a limb or other compressible external site takes precedence. This is followed by managing airway threats, ensuring adequate breathing, assessing circulatory status, disability, and exposing the body to allow a thorough evaluation.

- **X**—EXsanguinating hemorrhage
- **A**—Airway
- **B**—Breathing
- **C**—Circulation
- **D**—Disability
- **E**—Expose/Environment

QUICK TIP

When correcting immediate life-threatening bleeding:

- Locate the source of bleeding.
  - Apply pressure to the source until bleeding stops.
- Use hemostatic dressings or tourniquets to stop bleeding.
- Avoid "popping the clot" and further diluting the blood through fluid resuscitation.
- Remember, all red blood cells count!

PHTLS—Past, Present, Future

Past

As often happens, a personal experience brought about the changes in emergency care that resulted in the Advanced Trauma Life Support (ATLS) course, and, eventually, the PHTLS program. ATLS started in 1978, 2 years after a private plane crash in a rural area of Nebraska, where an orthopedic surgeon's wife was killed, and his children were critically injured. The surgeon recognized the lack of a trauma care delivery system to treat acutely injured patients in rural settings. He and his colleagues decided that rural physicians needed to be trained in a systematic manner on treating trauma patients. They chose to use a format similar to Advanced Cardiovascular Life Support (ACLS) and called it Advanced Trauma Life Support. The ATLS course, developed and revised by the American College of Surgeons Committee on Trauma (ACS COT), is the basis of PHTLS.

Present

The first chairman of the ATLS ad hoc committee for the American College of Surgeons (ACS) and Chairman of the Prehospital Care Subcommittee on Trauma for the American College of Surgeons, Dr. Norman E. McSwain, Jr., FACS, knew that ATLS would have a profound effect on the outcomes of trauma patients. Moreover, he had a strong sense that an even greater effect could come from bringing this type of critical training to prehospital care providers.

Dr. McSwain, a founding member of the board of directors of the National Association of Emergency Medical Technicians (NAEMT), put together the draft curriculum of what would become PHTLS. With this curriculum in place, a committee was established in 1983. This committee continued to refine the curriculum and later that same year, pilot courses were launched in Louisiana, Iowa, and Connecticut.

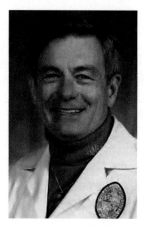

Figure 1-5 Dr. Norman E. McSwain, Jr., helped transform prehospital trauma care.
Courtesy Norman McSwain, MD, FACS, NREMT-P.

Strong Partnerships Make Good Providers

Throughout the growth of PHTLS, medical oversight has been provided through the ACS COT. For over 30 years, the partnership between the ACS and NAEMT has ensured that PHTLS course participants receive the opportunity to give trauma patients their best chance at survival.

Vision for the Future

The PHTLS program brings together the work of practitioners and researchers around the globe to determine standards of trauma care for the new millennium. PHTLS is currently taught in over 69 countries worldwide (for a current list of countries see: www.naemt.org/education/naemt-education-worldwide)

The Future Looks Bright

As prehospital trauma care evolves and improves, so too must the PHTLS program. We are dedicated to ongoing evaluation of the program to identify and implement improvements wherever needed. We will pursue new methods and technology for delivering PHTLS to enhance the clinical and service quality of the program.

FOR MORE INFORMATION

Refer to the "PHTLS—Past, Present, Future" section of Chapter 1: PHTLS: Past, Present, and Future.

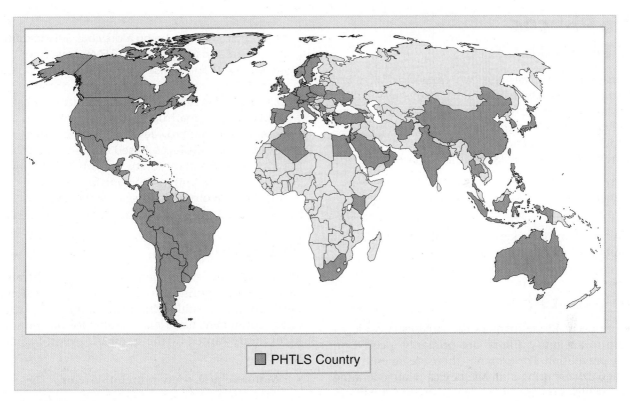

PHTLS Country

Figure 1-6 PHTLS is taught across the globe.

© Jones & Bartlett Learning.

Principles and Preferences

The science of medicine provides the principles of medical care. Simply stated, *principles* define the duties required of the prehospital care provider in optimizing patient survival and outcome. How these principles are implemented to most efficiently manage the patient depends on the *preferences*, which describe how a system and its individual providers choose to apply scientific principles to the care of patients. Let us take airway management, for example:

- The *principle* is that air, containing oxygen, must be moved through an open airway into the alveoli of the lungs to facilitate oxygen–carbon dioxide exchange with red blood cells (RBCs) so they may deliver oxygen to other tissues.
- The *preference* is how airway management is implemented in a particular patient. In some cases, patients will manage their own airway; in other patients, the prehospital care provider will have to decide which adjunct is best to facilitate airway management. In other words, the provider will determine the best method to ensure that the air passages are open to get oxygen into the lungs and, secondarily, to get carbon dioxide out.

QUICK TIP

Keep in mind that there are standards of care that everyone must follow in applying scientific principles to the care of individual patients.

CRITICAL-THINKING QUESTION

Can you think of a time when you had to employ a principle over your own preference?

The foundation of PHTLS is to teach prehospital care providers to make appropriate decisions for patient care based on knowledge, not on protocol. The goal of patient care is to achieve the principle. How this is achieved (i.e., the decision made by the provider to manage the patient) is the preference based on the situation, patient condition, fund of knowledge and skill, local protocols, and equipment available at the time.

FOR MORE INFORMATION

Refer to the "Principles and Preferences" section of Chapter 2: Golden Principles, Preferences, and Critical Thinking.

The Phases of Trauma Care

Traumatic incidents fall into two categories: *intentional* and *unintentional*. Intentional injury results from an act carried out on purpose with the goal of harming, injuring, or killing. Traumatic injury that occurs as an unintended or accidental consequence is considered unintentional.

Trauma care is divided into three phases:

- Pre-event
- Event
- Postevent

Actions can be taken to minimize the impact of traumatic injury during any of these three phases. You have critical responsibilities during each phase.

Pre-event Phase

The pre-event phase involves the circumstances leading up to an injury. Efforts are primarily focused on injury prevention. For example, there are an estimated 660,000 drivers using a mobile device while operating motor vehicles on any given day. Distracted driving in 2015 led to 3,500 deaths and 400,000 injuries in the United States. Prevention efforts have taken place to curb this rising trend, such as legal enforcement aimed specifically at preventing traffic accidents. To achieve maximum effect, strategies in the pre-event phase should focus on the most significant contributors to mortality and morbidity.

As a prehospital care provider, you need to prepare for events that are not preventable by:

- Maintaining your education on the most current evidence-based medical practices
- Updating your medical knowledge (much like you update your handheld devices)
- Reviewing new and current equipment on your response unit at the beginning of your shift and in trainings
- Understanding individual responsibilities and expectations of shift and patient care duties
- Understanding how to make the best use of your environment and your resources (e.g., roads, hospitals)

Safety Programs: Breaking the Fall

Promoting programs that raise awareness among populations at risk for falling is an area of significant public health effort. Prehospital care providers are in a unique position to play a role in fall prevention. With one of the leading risk factors for a fall resulting in injury or death among older adults being a previous fall incident, it is entirely possible that local EMS personnel are encountering at-risk individuals during calls for lift assistance or minor injury. These calls present an important opportunity for local public safety departments to collaborate with other healthcare providers and organizations to develop an evidence-based fall prevention program in the community. See NAEMT's Injury and Illness Prevention webpage for resources: http://naemt.org/initiatives/prevention.

Event Phase

The event phase is the moment of the actual trauma. Actions taken during this phase are aimed at minimizing injury resulting from the trauma. The use of safety equipment has a major influence on the severity of injury caused by the traumatic event. Examples include:

- Motor vehicle safety restraint systems
- Air bags
- Motorcycle helmets
- Child safety seats

Fix It and Click It

Many trauma centers, law enforcement organizations, and EMS and fire systems conduct programs to educate parents on the correct installation and use of child safety seats. When correctly installed and properly used, child safety seats offer infants and children the best protection during the event phase of trauma care.

Whether driving a personal vehicle or an emergency vehicle, you need to protect yourself and teach by example. You are responsible for yourself, your partner, and the patients under your care while in your ambulance or vehicle. It is your responsibility to prevent injury by safe and attentive driving.

QUICK TIP

The same level of attention you give to your patient care must be given to your driving. Always use the personal protective devices available, such as vehicle restraints, in the driving compartment and in the passenger or patient care compartment.

Postevent Phase

The postevent phase deals with the outcome of the traumatic event. Obviously, the worst possible outcome is death of the patient. These deaths can be prevented and outcomes in trauma patients improved by good prehospital care and hospital care, including:

- Early and aggressive management of shock
- Aggressive hemorrhage control
- Damage control resuscitation in the hospital

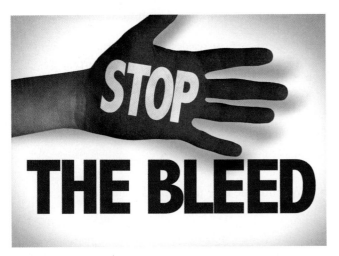

Figure 1-7 Immediate deaths can be prevented by injury prevention strategies and public education programs. Early deaths can be prevented through timely, appropriate prehospital care to reduce mortality and morbidity. Late deaths can be prevented only through prompt transport to a hospital appropriately staffed for trauma care.

© Gustavo Frazao/Shutterstock.

One of your most important responsibilities as a prehospital care provider is to spend as little time on the scene as possible and expedite your field care and transport of the patient. Studies show that the time from injury to arrival at the appropriate trauma center is critical to survival.

Golden Period—How Much Time Does a Patient Have?

In the late 1960s, R Adams Cowley, MD, conceived the idea of a crucial time period during which it is important to begin definitive patient care for a critically injured trauma patient. This time period came to be known as the "Golden Hour." The "hour" was intended to be figurative and not a literal description of a period of time. A patient with a penetrating wound to the heart may have only a few minutes to reach definitive care before shock becomes irreversible, but a patient with slow, ongoing internal hemorrhage from an isolated fracture may have several hours or longer to reach definitive care and resuscitation.

Because the Golden Hour is not a strict 60-minute time frame and varies from patient to patient based on the injuries, we often use the term *Golden Period*. The ACS COT has used this concept to emphasize the importance of transporting trauma patients to facilities where expert trauma care is available in a timely manner.

Golden Period—Critical Timing!

Some patients have less than an hour in which to receive care, whereas others have more time. In many urban prehospital systems in the United States, the average time between activation of EMS and arrival to the scene is 8 to 9 minutes, not including the time between injury and the call to the public safety answering point. A typical transport time to the receiving facility is another 8 to 9 minutes. If the prehospital care providers spend only 10 minutes on the scene, over 30 minutes of time will have already passed by the time a patient arrives at the receiving facility. Every additional minute spent on the scene is additional time that the patient is bleeding, and valuable time is ticking away from the Golden Period.

CRITICAL-THINKING QUESTION

What is the average on-scene time in your service?

One of the most important responsibilities of a prehospital care provider is to expedite the field care and transport of the patient. In the 2000s, prehospital scene times have decreased by allowing all providers (fire, police, and EMS) to work as a cohesive team by using a standard methodology across emergency services. As a result, patient survival has increased.

A second responsibility is transporting the patient to an appropriate facility. A factor that is extremely critical to a compromised patient's survival is the length of time that elapses between the incident and the provision of definitive care. Trauma center designations are developed at local or state levels, and the regulations for what resources must be available for each category of trauma center (level I, level II, level III, etc.) vary from state to state. The ACS evaluates trauma centers to verify the presence of resources listed in the ACS document: *Resources for Optimal Care of the Injured Patient.* A description of the different levels of trauma centers can be found on the Brain Trauma Foundation's website: https://braintrauma.org/news/article/trauma-center-designations.

FOR MORE INFORMATION

Refer to "The Phases of Trauma Care" section of Chapter 1: PHTLS: Past, Present, and Future.

Communication and Documentation

Communication about a trauma patient with the receiving hospital involves three components:

- Prearrival warning
- Verbal report upon arrival
- Written documentation of the encounter in the patient care report (PCR)

Care of the trauma patient is a team effort. The response to a critical trauma patient begins with the prehospital care provider and continues in the hospital. Delivering information from the prehospital setting to the receiving hospital allows for notification and mobilization of appropriate hospital resources to ensure an optimal reception of the patient.

Write It Down

Effective documentation, as provided in the PCR, fulfills several key functions:

- Maintains continuity of high-quality patient care
- Documents the assessment and management of the patient in the field for legal purposes
- Supports and continues trauma research
- Supports trauma system funding

LESSON WRAP-UP

- We must critically examine how and why we do everything.
- Science is always evolving, helping us to verify or refute our approach to trauma care.
- We must be able to adapt to changes.

STUDY QUESTIONS

1. In general, what is the leading cause of death in the United States?
   A. Intentional injury
   B. Unintentional injury
   C. Heart disease
   D. Cancer

2. Actions taken during the event phase of trauma care are designed to:
   A. educate the public on safety strategies.
   B. minimize the injury.
   C. prevent the injury.
   D. deal with injury resulting from the trauma.

3. Which of the following does PHTLS *not* provide?
   A. Understanding of anatomy and physiology of trauma

   B. The assessment of a trauma patient using the XABCDE approach
   C. The skills needed to provide care to a trauma patient
   D. Specific care protocols for different classes of trauma patients

4. Which of the following is a key change in the PHTLS recommendations for the assessment and treatment of trauma patients?
   A. American Heart Association (AHA) revised CPR guidelines
   B. Pediatric intubation
   C. XABCDE
   D. American College of Cardiology (ACC) blood pressure guidelines

ANSWER KEY

Question 1: B
Unintentional injury is the leading cause of death in people between 1 and 45 years of age. Worldwide, over 5 million people die annually as a result of injury, accounting for 9% of deaths.

Question 2: B
The event phase is the moment of the actual trauma. Actions taken during the event phase are aimed at minimizing injury as the result of the trauma.

Question 3: D

PHTLS provides an understanding of anatomy and physiology, the pathophysiology of trauma, the assessment and care of the trauma patient using the XABCDE approach, and the skills needed to provide that care—no more and no less. PHTLS neither recommends nor prohibits specific actions for the prehospital care provider.

Question 4: C

The new focus is on using the XABCDE approach to patient assessment.

REFERENCES AND FURTHER READING

American College of Surgeons. Resources for optimal care of the injured patient. https://www.facs.org/~/media/files/quality%20programs/trauma/vrc%20resources/resources%20for%20optimal%20care.ashx. Published 2014. Accessed October 18, 2018.

Brain Trauma Foundation. Trauma center designations and levels. https://braintrauma.org/news/article/trauma-center-designations. Published January 1, 2000. Accessed October 18, 2018.

National Association of Emergency Medical Technicians. *PHTLS: Prehospital Trauma Life Support.* 9th ed. Burlington, MA: Public Safety Group; 2019.

National Association of Emergency Medical Technicians. Injury and illness prevention. http://naemt.org/initiatives/prevention. Last updated 2018. Accessed October 18, 2018.

National Safety Council. Injury facts: societal costs. https://injuryfacts.nsc.org/all-injuries/costs/societal-costs/. Published 2017. Accessed October 18, 2018.

LESSON 2

Scene Management and Primary Survey

LESSON OBJECTIVES
- Identify scene safety threats posing a hazard to personnel, patients, and bystanders.
- Develop a patient approach plan using information gathered during a scene size-up.
- Describe the integration of assessment and management during the primary survey.
- Apply a Model Uniform Core Criteria (MUCC)-compliant triage method to manage multiple casualty incidents.
- Identify indications of intimate partner violence.

Introduction

There are a number of concerns you must be aware of when responding to a call and arriving on scene. The information gathered by the dispatch center is critical, not only for your safety, but for that of everyone in the general area. Your assessment of the scene is a continuous event that must come with a plan of action if the need to evacuate arises.

The on-scene information-gathering process begins immediately upon arrival at the incident. Before approaching the patient, evaluate the scene by:

PROGRESSIVE CASE STUDY: PART 1

You are dispatched to a small industrial site for a person trapped in one of the machines in the building. The patient is a 34-year-old male with his right leg caught in an industrial machine. Your ambulance is dispatched along with fire apparatus carrying extrication tools.

A small tertiary hospital is 15 minutes away by ground. A level 1 trauma center is 45 minutes away by ground and 10 minutes by air; a helicopter is 25 minutes from the scene.

Question:
- What scene safety concerns or considerations are present?

1. Obtaining a general impression of the situation for scene safety
2. Looking at the cause and results of the incident
3. Observing family members and bystanders

The appearance of the scene influences the entire assessment. You can gather a wealth of information by simply looking, listening, and cataloguing as much information as possible, including the mechanism of injury (MOI), the present situation, and the overall degree of safety.

Scene Size-Up

The first consideration when approaching any scene is the safety of *all* emergency responders. When emergency medical services (EMS) personnel become victims, not only can they no longer assist others, they add to the number of patients. Patient care may need to wait until the scene is safe enough for you to enter without undue risk. Safety concerns should include:

- Exposure to body fluids
- Exposure to chemical weapons used in warfare
- Fire
- Downed electrical lines
- Explosives
- Hazardous materials
- Traffic
- Floodwater
- An assailant on scene
- Adverse weather conditions

Situation

Assessment of the situation follows the safety assessment. The situational survey includes issues that may affect how you manage the patient as well as incident-specific concerns related to the patient directly.

QUICK TIP

Questions you should consider when assessing the issues posed by a given situation include:

- What really happened at the scene? What were the circumstances that led to the injury? Was it intentional or unintentional?
- Why was help summoned, and who summoned it?
- What was the MOI? The majority of patient injuries can be predicted based on evaluating and understanding the kinematics involved in the incident.
- How many people are involved, and what are their ages?
- Are additional EMS units needed for scene management, patient treatment, or transport?
- Are any other personnel or resources needed (e.g., law enforcement, fire department, power company)?
- Is special extrication or rescue equipment needed?
- Is helicopter transport necessary?
- Is a physician needed to assist with triage or on-scene medical care issues?
- Could a medical problem be the instigating factor that led to the trauma (e.g., a vehicle collision that resulted from the driver's heart attack or stroke)?

Predicting Patient Injuries Based on the MOI

The information you gather from your scene size-up allows you and your team to forecast the injuries your patient may have suffered. The saying "a picture is worth a thousand words" holds true when dealing with an MOI. Your ability to obtain the critical information during the size-up and to pass that information along to the trauma center plays a profound role in patient outcome.

Issues related to safety and situation overlap significantly; many safety topics are also specific to certain situations, and certain situations pose serious safety hazards.

Forming a general impression of the patient within the first few moments of contact is critical. The primary survey of the trauma patient includes:

- **X** (eXsanguinating hemorrhage)—Identify severe external bleeding.
- **A** (Airway management and cervical spine stabilization)—Identify airway compromise or potential for this to develop.
- **B** (Breathing)—Identify breathing inadequacy or potential for this to develop.
- **C** (Circulation)—Identify hypoperfusion; control mild to moderate bleeding.
- **D** (Disability)—Identify neurologic dysfunction.
- **E** (Expose/environment)—Identify significant injuries.

This sequence protects the ability of the body to oxygenate and the ability of the red blood cells (RBCs) to deliver oxygen to the tissues.

PROGRESSIVE CASE STUDY: PART 2

A dispatched fire engine with a crew of four and extrication equipment arrives before your ambulance. The 34-year-old male has been removed from the machinery and is sitting against a wall. The fire crew reports the patient's right leg was pulled into exposed machinery up to the knee. There was no associated fall or any other injury.

The patient is in a large, well-lit room at a safe distance from the stopped and partially disassembled machine. He appears alert but is pale and diaphoretic. His right lower leg is wrapped in blood-soaked dressings, from which blood is dripping. There is a large amount of blood staining the patient's right pants leg and a blood trail from the machinery to a pool of blood beside him. The patient's right pants leg is torn, and the dressings are not controlling the bleeding. Estimated blood loss on scene is 1.5 liters.

Questions:

- What is the MOI?
- Is cervical spine motion restriction indicated by the MOI?
- Do you have enough resources to manage this patient?

QUICK TIP

When determining the MOI in the progressive case study, consider these questions:

- What protective equipment was used?
- How was the leg pulled into the machine?
- How was the leg removed?
- How much blood has been lost?
- How severe was the bleeding prior to bandaging?

FOR MORE INFORMATION

Refer to the "Scene Assessment" and "Safety Issues" sections of Chapter 5: Scene Management.

Patient Approach Plan

Once you have determined that the scene is safe, you can complete a rapid patient assessment. For the trauma patient, as for other critically ill patients, assessment is the foundation on which all management and transport decisions are based. You need to develop an overall impression of a patient's status and establish baseline values for the patient's respiratory, circulatory, and neurologic systems. When life-threatening conditions are identified, you need to immediately intervene. If time and the patient's condition allow, you will conduct a secondary survey for injuries that are not life- or limb-threatening. Often this secondary survey occurs during patient transport.

The primary survey must proceed rapidly and in a logical order. If you are alone, you can perform some key interventions as you identify life-threatening conditions. If more than one provider is present, one may complete the primary survey while others initiate

Different Populations, Same Survey

The same primary survey approach is utilized regardless of the patient type. All patients, including geriatric, pediatric, or pregnant patients, are assessed in a similar fashion to ensure that all components of the assessment are covered and that no significant pathology is missed.

care. When several critical conditions are identified, the primary survey allows you to establish treatment priorities. In general, you should manage compressible external hemorrhage first, an airway issue is managed before a breathing problem, and so forth. Each crew member going into the scene should have a plan for his or her responsibilities and how he or she will achieve them.

General Impression

The primary survey begins with a rapid global overview of the status of a patient's respiratory, circulatory, and neurologic systems to identify obvious threats, such as:

- Evidence of severe compressible hemorrhage
- Airway, breathing, or circulation compromise
- Gross deformities

When initially approaching a patient, look for severe compressible hemorrhage and check whether the patient appears to be moving air effectively, is awake or unresponsive, and is moving spontaneously. Once at the patient's side, introduce yourself to the patient and ask the patient's name. A reasonable next step is to ask the patient, "What happened to you?" If the patient

PROGRESSIVE CASE STUDY: PART 3

Your primary survey reveals the following:

- **X**—Uncontrolled severe external bleeding at right leg; controlled with tourniquet
- **A**—Airway patent
- **B**—Slow, deep breaths are adequate; provide supplemental oxygen
- **C**—Skin is pale and moist, radial pulse is rapid
- **D**—Glasgow coma scale (GCS) score: 15; absence of motor function, sensation, and pulse distal to injury site
- **E**—Right leg avulsed from the knee, open fracture of the tibia and femur

Questions:

- What are the potential life threats?
- What treatment technique is indicated for the patient in this case?
- If the patient was unresponsive and breathing was shallow and fast (> 30 breaths/minute), how would you initially manage the patient?

appears comfortable and can answer coherently in complete sentences, you can conclude that the patient has a patent airway, sufficient respiratory function to support speech, adequate cerebral perfusion, and reasonable neurologic functioning; there are probably no immediate threats to this patient's life.

If a patient cannot provide an answer or appears in distress, begin a detailed primary survey to identify life-threatening problems. You should be able to obtain a general impression of the patient's overall condition in a few seconds. This is also where your "gut feeling" comes into play and is something that with training and experience you should learn to rely on.

Managing Life Threats

Sick or Not Sick?

By rapidly assessing vital functions, the primary survey serves to establish whether the patient is presently or imminently critical.

In the critical multisystem trauma patient, the priority for care is the rapid identification and management of life-threatening conditions. The majority of trauma patients have injuries that involve only one system (such as an isolated limb fracture). For these trauma patients, there is often time for a more thorough primary survey and a secondary survey. For the critically injured patient, you may not be able to conduct more than a primary survey. In these critical patients, the emphasis is on rapid evaluation, initiation of resuscitation, and transport to an appropriate medical facility. The emphasis on rapid transport does not eliminate the need for prehospital treatment. Rather, treatment should be done faster and more efficiently and possibly started en route to the receiving facility.

Because quick establishment of priorities and the general impression and recognition of life-threatening injuries is critical, you should memorize the components of the primary and secondary surveys and understand and perform the logical progression of priority-based assessment and treatment the same way every time, regardless of the severity of the injury.

Know Your ABCs, CABs, and XABCDEs

Similar to Advanced Cardiovascular Life Support (ACLS), in which the priority of the primary survey has changed from ABC to CAB, the primary survey of the trauma patient now emphasizes

control of life-threatening external bleeding as the first step in the sequence. While the steps of the primary survey are taught and displayed in a sequential manner, many of the steps can—and should—be performed simultaneously. The steps can be remembered using the mnemonic XABCDE:

- **X**—eXsanguinating hemorrhage (control of severe external bleeding)
- **A**—Airway management and cervical spine stabilization
- **B**—Breathing (ventilation and oxygenation)
- **C**—Circulation (perfusion and other hemorrhage)
- **D**—Disability
- **E**—Expose/environment

Control of Severe External Bleeding

In the primary survey of a trauma patient, you must immediately identify and manage life-threatening external hemorrhage. If you are dealing with an exsanguinating external hemorrhage, it needs to be controlled even before assessing the airway or performing other interventions such as spinal immobilization. This type of bleeding typically involves arterial bleeding from an extremity, but it may also occur from the scalp or at the junction of an extremity with the trunk (junctional bleeding) and other sites.

When to Press and When to Pack

Direct pressure and hemostatic packing and dressings should be applied in cases of nonarterial severe bleeding in extremities and all severe bleeding from truncal sites.

Hemorrhage Control

External hemorrhage needs to be identified and controlled in the primary survey, because if it is not controlled as soon as possible, the potential for death increases dramatically. The three types of external hemorrhage are capillary, venous, and arterial.

Rapid control of bleeding is one of the most important goals in the care of a trauma patient. Nothing else can happen until external bleeding is controlled. Hemorrhage can be controlled in the following ways:

1. *Direct pressure*. Direct pressure is exactly what the name implies—applying pressure

to the site of bleeding. This is best accomplished by placing a dressing (e.g., hemostatic gauze is preferred) directly over the site of bleeding (if it can be identified) and applying pressure.

- Apply pressure as precisely and focally as possible. A gloved finger on a visible compressible artery is often very effective.
- Apply pressure continuously for a minimum of 3 minutes (or per the manufacturer's instructions for hemostatic gauze) and for 10 minutes if using plain gauze (this is the time required to form a clot).
- Avoid the temptation to remove pressure to check if the wound is still bleeding before that time period elapses.

The application and maintenance of direct pressure requires all of your attention, preventing you from participating in other aspects of patient care. Alternatively, or if assistance is limited, a pressure dressing can be applied. Remember that application of pressure is a simple move that can be administered by a bystander, if necessary, provided he or she has a pair of gloves.

2. *Tourniquets*. Tourniquets are very effective in controlling severe hemorrhage when direct pressure or a pressure dressing cannot control bleeding from an extremity or if there are not enough personnel available on scene to perform other bleeding control methods. In the case of life-threatening, or exsanguinating, hemorrhage, you should apply a tourniquet instead of or concurrent with other bleeding control measures (i.e., as a first-line treatment for this type of bleeding).

Tourniquets should be placed as proximal as possible (i.e., near the groin or axilla) on the affected limb. You can also use other bleeding control measures, such as direct pressure and hemostatic agents, but they should not delay or take the place of tourniquet placement on an injured limb with severe arterial bleeding.

Occasionally, bleeding from distal or smaller arteries can be controlled with focused direct compression of the artery. However, this should only be performed if such bleeding can be controlled with a rapidly applied pressure dressing or if there is enough help on scene so that one provider can maintain manual direct pressure.

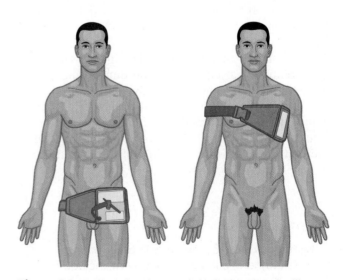

Figure 2-1 The junctional areas at the inguinal and axillae regions.

© Jones & Bartlett Learning.

If not, apply a tourniquet to the affected extremity. Severe bleeding from junctional areas may be managed by placing an appropriate junctional tourniquet, if available, or packing with hemostatic gauze and placing a pressure dressing.

Slow the Flow

Junctional hemorrhage is defined as bleeding that occurs where two anatomically distinct zones come together. Examples of junctional areas include:

- The lower abdomen
- Groin
- Axillae
- Proximal extremities

The use of a tourniquet or pressure dressing in these areas is often both impractical and ineffective.

QUICK TIP

The use of "elevation" and pressure on "pressure points" is no longer recommended because of insufficient data supporting their effectiveness.

Airway

Check the patient's airway quickly to ensure that it is patent (open and clear) and that there is no danger of obstruction. If the airway is compromised, it will need to be opened, initially using manual methods (trauma chin lift or trauma jaw thrust), and cleared of blood, body substances, and foreign bodies, if necessary.

Eventually, as equipment and time become available, airway management can advance to include suction and mechanical means (oral airway, nasal airway, supraglottic airways, and endotracheal intubation or transtracheal methods). However, a simple and quick method should always be used first to make sure the airway is open.

QUICK TIP

Numerous factors play a role in determining the method of airway management, including available equipment, the skill level of the prehospital care provider, and the distance from the trauma center.

Spinal Stabilization

You should suspect that every trauma patient with a significant blunt MOI has a spinal injury until it is conclusively ruled out. When establishing an open airway, consider the possibility of cervical spine injury. Excessive movement in any direction could either cause or aggravate neurologic damage. The solution is to ensure that the patient's head and neck are manually maintained (stabilized) in the neutral position during the entire assessment process, especially when opening the airway and administering necessary ventilation.

This does not mean that necessary airway maintenance procedures cannot be applied. Instead, it means that the procedures need to be performed while protecting the patient's spine from unnecessary movement. If you need to remove a spinal immobilization device that was placed beforehand in order to reassess the patient or perform an intervention, you need to apply manual stabilization of the head and neck until the patient can again be placed in spinal immobilization.

QUICK TIP

It is particularly important to maintain a high index of suspicion for spinal injury in elderly or chronically debilitated patients, even with more minor MOIs.

Breathing

Once the patient's airway is open, the quality and quantity of the patient's breathing (ventilation) can be evaluated:

1. Check to see if the patient is breathing by looking for chest motion and feeling for air movement from the mouth or nose. If uncertain, auscultate both sides of the chest to evaluate lung sounds.
2. If the patient is not breathing, immediately begin assisting ventilations (while maintaining cervical spine stabilization in a neutral position, when indicated) with a bag-mask device with supplemental oxygen before continuing the assessment.
3. Continue assisted ventilation, and prepare to insert an oral, nasal (if no severe facial trauma), or supraglottic airway (if no signs of severe oropharyngeal trauma); intubate; or provide

---

QUICK TIP

Do not allow an advanced airway procedure to increase your scene time. If the procedure can be accomplished in the back of the ambulance, perform it there.

other means of mechanical airway protection. Also, be prepared to suction blood, vomitus, or other fluids from the airway.

4. If the patient is breathing, estimate the adequacy of the ventilatory rate and depth to determine whether the patient is moving enough air (minute ventilation = rate × depth).

5. Ensure that the patient is not hypoxic and that the oxygen saturation is greater than or equal to 94%. Provide supplemental oxygen (and assisted ventilation) as needed to maintain an adequate oxygen saturation.

6. If the patient is conscious, listen to the patient talk to assess whether he or she can speak a full sentence without difficulty. Also note any airway sounds that you may hear as he or she speaks (i.e., raspy voice, stridor, wheezing).

It Takes Your Breath Away

Injuries that may impede ventilation include:

- Tension pneumothorax
- Flail chest
- Spinal cord injuries
- Traumatic brain injuries

These injuries should be identified or suspected during the primary survey and require that ventilatory support be initiated at once. Needle decompression should be performed immediately if tension pneumothorax is suspected.

Circulation

Assessing for circulatory system compromise or failure is the next step in caring for the trauma patient. Oxygenation of the RBCs without delivery to the tissue cells is of no benefit to the patient. After assessing the patient's airway and breathing status, you can get an adequate overall estimate of the patient's cardiac output and perfusion status. Hemorrhage—either external or internal—is the most common cause of preventable death from trauma. The patient's overall circulatory status can be determined by checking peripheral pulses and evaluating skin color, temperature, and moisture.

QUICK TIP

Assessment of perfusion may be challenging in geriatric or pediatric patients or in those who are well conditioned or taking certain medications (such as beta blockers). Shock in trauma patients is almost always due to external or internal hemorrhage.

The potential sites of massive internal hemorrhage include:

- The chest (both pleural cavities)
- The abdomen (peritoneal cavity)
- The pelvis
- The retroperitoneal space
- The extremities (primarily the thighs)

Bleeding in these areas is not easy to control outside the hospital. If available, apply a pelvic binder rapidly to potential "open book" pelvic injuries. The goal is rapid delivery of the patient to a facility equipped and appropriately staffed for rapid control of hemorrhage in the operating room (i.e., a trauma center).

Evaluate the pulse for presence, quality, and regularity. A quick check of the pulse will reveal whether the patient has tachycardia, bradycardia, or an irregular rhythm.

Feel the Beat

While the absence of peripheral pulses in the presence of central pulses usually represents profound hypotension, the presence of peripheral pulses should not be overly reassuring.

In the primary survey, determination of an exact pulse rate is not necessary. Instead, quickly get a rough estimate, and obtain the actual pulse rate later in the process. In trauma patients, it is important to consider treatable causes of abnormal vital signs and physical findings.

CAUTION

Pulse Pressure Association

In the past, the presence of a radial pulse was thought to indicate a systolic blood pressure of at least 80 mm Hg, with the presence of a femoral pulse indicating blood pressure of at least 70 mm Hg, and presence of only a carotid pulse indicating blood pressure of 60 mm Hg. Evidence has shown this theory to be inaccurate; it actually overestimates blood pressures. It can, however, be considered a good assessment of peripheral perfusion.

Disability

The next step in the primary survey is assessment of nervous system function (including spinal cord). This begins with determining the patient's level of consciousness (LOC).

You should assume that a confused, belligerent, combative, or uncooperative patient is hypoxic or has suffered a traumatic brain injury (TBI) until proved otherwise. Most patients want help when their lives are medically threatened. If a patient refuses help, you need to consider why. Does the patient feel threatened? If so, further attempts to establish rapport can help gain the patient's trust. If nothing in the situation seems to be threatening, the source of the behavior may be physiologic, and reversible conditions need to be identified and treated.

During the assessment, the history can help determine whether the patient lost consciousness at any time since the injury occurred, whether toxic substances might be involved (and what they might be), and whether the patient has any preexisting conditions that may produce a decreased LOC or aberrant behavior. Careful observation of the scene can provide invaluable information in this regard.

A decreased LOC should alert you to the following possibilities:

- Decreased cerebral oxygenation (caused by hypoxia/hypoperfusion) or severe hypoventilation (CO_2 narcosis)
- Central nervous system (CNS) injury (e.g., TBI)
- Drug or alcohol overdose or toxin exposure
- Metabolic derangement (e.g., caused by diabetes, seizure, or cardiac arrest)

QUICK TIP

Recent research has found that using only the motor component of the GCS, and specifically, if this component is less than 6 (meaning the patient does not follow commands), is just as predictive for severe injury as using the whole GCS.

If a patient is not awake, oriented, or able to follow commands, quickly assess spontaneous extremity movement as well as the patient's pupils.

- Are the pupils equal and round, reactive to light (PERRLA)?
- Are the pupils equal to each other? Is each pupil round and of normal appearance?
- Does it appropriately react to light by constricting, or is it unresponsive and dilated?

A GCS score of less than 14 in combination with an abnormal pupil examination can indicate the presence of a life-threatening TBI.

Quickly check the movements of the four extremities as they can provide very important materializing signs of injury. Do not miss a gross hemiplegia or paraplegia at this stage, as it has important consequences on spinal management.

Expose/Environment

An early step in the assessment process is to remove a patient's clothes, because exposure of the trauma patient is critical to finding all injuries.

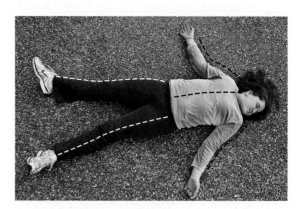

Figure 2-2 Clothing can be quickly removed by cutting, as indicated by the dotted lines.
© National Association of Emergency Medical Technicians.

You Can't Treat What You Don't See

The saying, "The one part of the body that is not exposed will be the most severely injured part," may not always be true, but it is true often enough to warrant a total body examination. Also, blood can collect in and be absorbed by clothing and go unnoticed. After seeing the patient's entire body, you can then cover the patient again to conserve body heat.

Although it is important to expose a trauma patient's body to complete an effective assessment, hypothermia is a serious problem in the management of a trauma patient. Only what is necessary should be exposed to the outside environment. Once the patient has been moved inside the warm ambulance, you can do a complete assessment and then cover the patient again as quickly as possible.

QUICK TIP

Take special care when cutting and removing clothing from a victim of a crime so as not to inadvertently destroy evidence.

FOR MORE INFORMATION

Refer to the "Primary Survey" section of Chapter 6: Patient Assessment and Management.

Transport

If life-threatening conditions are identified during the primary survey, the patient should be rapidly packaged after initiating limited field intervention. Initiate transport of critically injured trauma patients to the closest appropriate facility as soon as possible.

Limited scene time and initiation of rapid transport to the closest appropriate facility—preferably a trauma center—are fundamental aspects of prehospital trauma resuscitation.

Timing Is Everything

Keep scene time as brief as possible (ideally 10 minutes or less) when any of the following life-threatening conditions are present:

1. Inadequate or threatened airway
2. Impaired ventilation, as demonstrated by the following:
   - Abnormally fast or slow ventilatory rate
   - Hypoxia (Spo$_2$ < 94% even with supplemental oxygen)
   - Dyspnea
   - Open pneumothorax or flail chest
   - Suspected closed or tension pneumothorax
3. Significant external hemorrhage or suspected internal hemorrhage
4. Abnormal neurologic status
   - GCS score ≤ 13 or motor component < 6
   - Seizure activity
   - Sensory or motor deficit
5. Penetrating trauma to the head, neck, or torso or proximal to the elbow or knee in the extremities
6. Amputation or near-amputation proximal to the fingers or toes
7. Any significant trauma in the presence of the following:
   - History of serious medical conditions (e.g., coronary artery disease, chronic obstructive pulmonary disease, bleeding disorder)
   - Age > 55 years

- Hypothermia
- Burns
- Pregnancy

FOR MORE INFORMATION

Refer to the "Resuscitation" section of Chapter 6: Patient Assessment and Management.

Mass-Casualty Triage

A disaster is defined as a situation in which the number of patients presenting for medical assistance exceeds the capacity of healthcare providers with the usual resources at hand and requires additional, and sometimes external, assistance. This concept applies to all medical care settings, including hospitals and prehospital settings. This situation is commonly referred to as a mass-casualty incident (MCI).

QUICK TIP

The abbreviation MCI has also been used to refer to "multiple-casualty incidents," which are events that involve more than one casualty but may be handled with standard local resources.

When presented with such a situation, being able to effectively triage, treat, and transport patients in a timely manner can become overwhelming, so guidelines have been developed to aid in this process.

Triage is one of the most important missions of any disaster medical response. This usually means finding

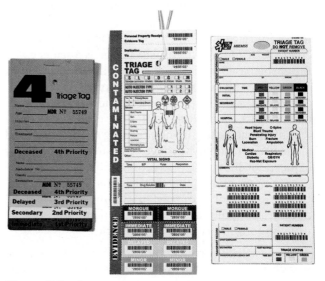

Figure 2-3 Triage tags.
© File of Life Foundation, Inc.

and treating the sickest patient. The objective of mass-casualty triage is to do the greatest good for the greatest number of people.

> **Corralling the Chaos**
>
> Mass-casualty triage in the field should be overseen by a trained triage officer. A triage officer should have a wide breadth of clinical experience in the assessment and management of field injuries, as potentially challenging decisions may be made about patients who are deemed critical versus those classified as mortally wounded or expectant.

START Triage

A number of different methodologies exist for evaluating and assigning the triage category. One method, the START triage algorithm (**s**imple **t**riage **a**nd **r**apid **t**reatment), involves a rapid physiologic and mental status evaluation. This system evaluates the respiratory status, perfusion status, and mental status of the patient in prioritizing casualties for immediate management.

> **QUICK TIP**
>
> Other triage systems include the MASS (**m**ove, **a**ssess, **s**ort, **s**end), Smart, JumpStart (pediatric algorithm), and Sacco triage methods.

SALT Triage

In an effort to provide national guidance and bring uniformity to the triage process, the U.S. Centers for Disease Control and Prevention (CDC) convened a multidisciplinary group of experts to develop a consensus-based triage system. The Model Uniform Core Criteria (MUCC) for Mass Casualty Triage is a science and consensus-based national guideline that recommends 24 core criteria for all mass-casualty triage systems, now known as SALT (Sort, Assess, Lifesaving interventions, and Treatment/transport).

This triage system involves sorting the patient based on the patient's ability to move, assessing the patient for the need for **l**ifesaving interventions, performing those interventions, and ultimately **t**reatment and **t**ransport.

Regardless of the exact triage method used, all triage systems ultimately classify patients into one of (usually) four injury-severity categories:

- Highest priority patients are those who are identified as having critical, but likely survivable, injuries and are usually categorized as *immediate* and color-coded *red*.

- Patients with non-life-threatening injuries (who may be nonambulatory) and can potentially tolerate a short delay in care are categorized as *delayed* patients and color-coded *yellow*.
- Patients with relatively minor injuries, often referred to as the "walking wounded," are classified as *minimal* victims and color-coded *green*.
- Patients who have expired on the scene or whose injuries are so severe that death is inevitable are categorized as *dead* or *expectant*, respectively, and color-coded *black*.

> **QUICK TIP**
>
> Some triage systems, particularly SALT, specifically separate those patients classified as mortally wounded from those who are dead, color coding the expectant as *gray* (the rationale here being that expectant care does not mean no care).

It is important that triage personnel avoid the temptation to pause triage in favor of treating a critically injured patient. During this initial triage phase, medical interventions are limited to those actions that are performed easily and rapidly, and are not labor intensive. Generally, this means performing only procedures such as:

- Manual airway opening
- Needle chest decompression
- Administration of a chemical antidote
- External hemorrhage control including wound packing and tourniquet deployment

Interventions such as bag-mask ventilation, closed chest compression, establishing IV access, and endotracheal intubation are often deferred during the triage process. As a general rule, any intervention that immobilizes the provider should be avoided.

> **FOR MORE INFORMATION**
>
> Refer to the "Patient Assessment and Triage" section of Chapter 5: Scene Management.

Violence

Every call has the potential to take you into an emotionally charged environment. Even a scene that appears safe has the potential to deteriorate quickly, so always be alert to subtle clues that suggest a change in the situation. The patient, family, or bystanders on

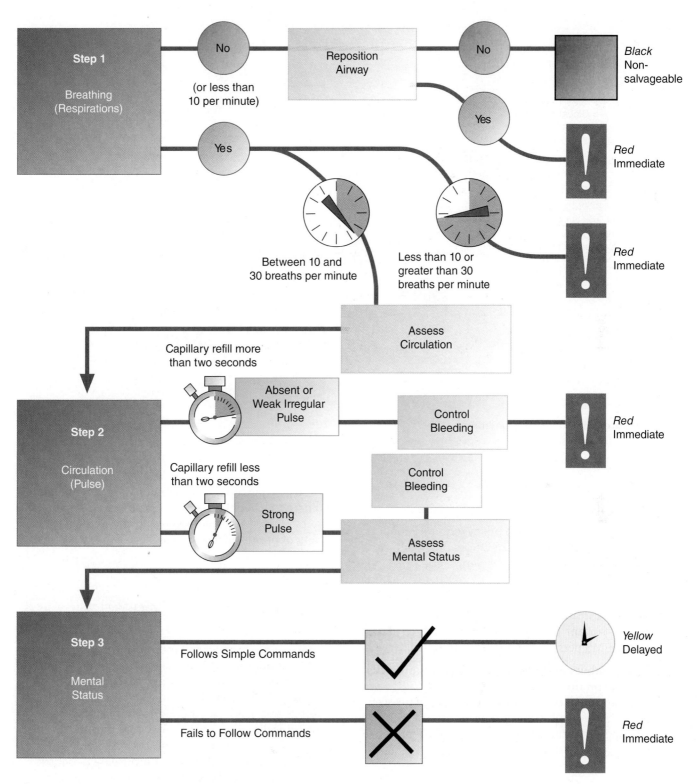

Figure 2-4 START triage algorithm: decision map.

Courtesy of Hoag Hospital Newport Beach and the Newport Beach Fire Department.

the scene may not be able to perceive the situation rationally. They may think the response time was too long, be overly sensitive to words or actions, and misunderstand the "usual" approach to patient assessment.

Maintaining a confident and professional manner while demonstrating respect and concern is important to gaining the patient's trust and achieving control of the scene.

SALT Mass Casualty Triage

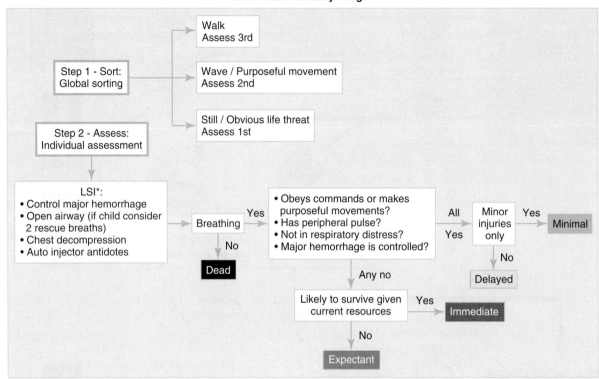

Figure 2-5 SALT triage algorithm.

Chemical Hazards Emergency Medical Management, U.S. Department of Health and Human Services. http://chemm.nlm.nih.gov/chemmimages/salt.png. Accessed October 16, 2017.

Know Before You Go

Some EMS agencies have a policy requiring the presence of law enforcement before providers enter a violent or potentially violent scene.

It is important for you to train yourself to *observe* the scene. EMS personnel must learn to notice:

- The numbers and locations of individuals when arriving on the scene
- The movement of bystanders into or out of the scene
- Any indicators of stress or tension
- Unexpected or unusual reactions to EMS presence

Be Aware!

Watch the patient's and bystanders' hands. Look for unusual bulges in waistbands, clothing that is worn out of season, or oversized clothing that could easily hide a weapon.

If you perceive a developing threat, immediately prepare to leave the scene. An assessment or a procedure may need to be completed in the ambulance. The safety of prehospital care providers is the first priority.

CRITICAL-THINKING QUESTION

Consider the following situation: You and your partner are in the living room of a patient's home. While your partner is checking the patient's blood pressure, an apparently intoxicated man enters the room from the back of the house. He looks angry, and you notice what appears to be the handle of a gun sticking out of the waistband of his pants. Your partner does not see or hear this person enter the room because he is focused on the patient. The suspicious person begins to question your presence and is extremely agitated about your uniform and your badge. His hands repeatedly move toward, then away from, his waist. He begins to pace and mumble. How can you and your partner prepare for this sort of situation?

Intimate Partner Violence

Intimate partner violence (IPV; commonly called domestic violence) occurs daily to individuals regardless of their age, sex, economic status, race, sexual orientation, or education. In the United States, a reported 1.3 million women and 835,000 men are involved in an IPV event annually. These events create physical and emotional injuries that sometimes take years to overcome. As a prehospital care provider, you may be placed into a situation where it is obvious that a hazard is present, but sometimes it is not so obvious.

Intimate Partner Violence

According to the CDC, IPV describes physical, sexual, or psychological harm by a current or former partner or spouse. This type of violence can occur among heterosexual or same-sex couples and does not require sexual intimacy.

Recognition of IPV is imperative in EMS. There are four predominant types of IPV:

- Physical violence, which is the intentional use of force to cause harm.
- Sexual violence, which can be further divided into five categories:
  - Rape
  - Victim made to penetrate someone else
  - Non-physically pressured unwanted penetration
  - Unwanted sexual contact
  - Non-contact unwanted sexual experiences
- Stalking
- Physical aggression

Read the Signs

Victims often suffer in silence due to the fear and control the abuser has over them. You must be able to recognize some of the signs that abuse is occurring, including:

- Overly timid patients—Does the patient avoid making eye contact with you or the partner, does the patient defer to the partner to answer questions?
- Overly protective partners—Do you notice that the patient's partner will not leave the patient alone with you?
- Unexplained or strange injuries—Does the patient's injury not match the patient's story?

- Belittling the patient—Do you notice the patient's partner putting down or humiliating the patient?
- Patient assessment—Are there signs of eating disturbances, anxiousness, depression, sleep problems, or hopelessness from the patient during the patient assessment?

As with any potentially violent scene, you must be aware of your surroundings. You may be stepping into an escalating situation where one party may not know you have been called, which can enrage the other partner. While on scene, watch the body movements and evaluate the moods of those in the situation. Ask if there are other people in the house that you may not see upon your initial entry. If the answer is yes, heighten your observation skills, listen for others, have your partner keep an eye out for others who have not presented themselves yet, and be ready to retreat if needed.

Be sure to document your findings when you believe that violence has occurred. Preserve any evidence that you may encounter as part of the patient assessment as you would with any other crime scene. It is critical that you understand your local laws on mandatory reporting of IPV and that your documentation is descriptive and sensitive to the situation.

Managing the Violent Scene

Partners need to discuss and agree on methods to handle a violent patient or bystander. Attempting to develop a process during the event is prone to failure. Partners can use a hands-on or hands-off approach, as well as predetermined code words and hand signals, for emergencies.

If both providers have all of their attention focused on the patient, the scene can quickly become threatening, and early clues may be missed. In many situations, patient, family, and bystander tension and anxiety are immediately reduced when one attentive provider begins interacting with and assessing the patient, while the other provider observes the scene.

Safety Strategies

There are various methods for dealing with a scene that has become dangerous, including the following:

1. *Don't be there.* When responding to a known violent scene, stage at a safe location until the scene has been rendered safe by law enforcement and clearance to respond has been given.

2. *Retreat.* If threats are presented when approaching the scene, tactfully retreat to the vehicle and leave the scene. Stage at a safe location and notify appropriate personnel.
3. *Defuse.* If a scene becomes threatening during patient care, use verbal skills to reduce tension and aggression (while preparing to leave the scene).
4. *Defend.* As a last resort, prehospital care providers may find it necessary to defend themselves. It is important that such efforts are to "disengage and get away." Do not attempt to chase or subdue an aggressive party. Ensure that law enforcement personnel have been notified and are en route. Again, the safety of the providers is the priority.

FOR MORE INFORMATION

Refer to the "Violence" section of Chapter 5: Scene Management.

PROGRESSIVE CASE STUDY: SUMMARY

The primary survey was completed and all life threats managed. The EMS unit met the helicopter, where the patient was transported to a level I trauma center and admitted for surgical treatment.

The patient was discharged 1 week later to a rehabilitation unit after an above-knee amputation of the right leg.

Critical Actions:

- External hemorrhage control using tourniquet to proximal thigh at groin
- Supplemental oxygen to avoid hypoxia
- Cover patient with blanket
- IV fluid administration to support perfusion

LESSON WRAP-UP

- Scene safety of prehospital care providers and the patient is the priority.
- All life threats are to be managed as soon as discovered.
- Maintain a high index of suspicion for subtle life-threatening injuries.

PROGRESSIVE CASE STUDY RECAP

Part 1	
What scene safety concerns or considerations are present?	Consider the scene in this case: ■ Is the machinery still operating or operational? ■ Are there nearby machines or equipment that is still operating that could risk personal safety? ■ Has there been an associated spillage of hazardous material (i.e., toxic, slip hazard, flammable, etc.)? ■ Is the environment safe (i.e., fumes, noise, level surfaces, trip hazards, confined space, fire/explosion risk)? ■ Is the machinery stable and safe to approach? ■ How many workers have been injured? Are all other workers accounted for? ■ Do you have sufficient resources to respond to this incident to address scene safety issues?

Part 2	
What is the MOI?	Consider the following: ■ What protective equipment was used (i.e., helmet, gloves, etc.)? ■ How was the leg pulled into the machine (i.e., did he fall into the machine, associated joint or muscle injuries, etc.)? ■ How was the leg removed (i.e., pulled out, or was the machine removed from around the leg)? ■ How much blood has been lost (i.e., was the bleeding severe while trapped or was it tamponaded or tourniqueted by the machine, etc.)? ■ How severe was the bleeding prior to bandaging (i.e., free flow or pulsatile flow, etc.)?
Is cervical spine motion restriction indicated by the MOI?	MOI does not suggest the need for cervical spine motion restriction.
Do you have enough resources to manage this patient?	Take into consideration whether there is any indication for launching a helicopter to assist with transport.

Part 3	
What are the potential life threats?	Exsanguinating hemorrhage

What treatment technique is indicated for the patient in this case?	1. External hemorrhage control in the form of:
	   · Direct pressure
	   · Tourniquet
	2. Provide supplemental oxygen to avoid hypoxia secondary to blood loss or loss of RBCs.
	3. Splinting and bandaging are important, even on the lactic acidosis syndrome (LAS) level to avoid further injury to blood vessels and/or nerves. Proper splinting is often overlooked in patient management and outcomes. Proper splinting can make the difference as to whether the patient has permanent damage and effects from the injury.

If the patient was unresponsive and breathing shallow and fast (> 30 breaths/minute), how would you initially manage the patient?	Manage all life threats first. ■ The patient can be managed simultaneously with multiple rescuers. ■ Manage uncontrolled arterial bleeding from the right leg with direct pressure and tourniquet. ■ Airway adjunct placed and ventilation with a bag-mask device at 12 breaths/min started to achieve proper tidal volume. ■ Secure the airway with an advanced airway prior to transport.

Part 4	
Where should this patient be transported?	The patient has a mangled and pulseless limb requiring rapid transport to a level I trauma center.
How should this patient be transported?	Helicopter transport is faster even if it is launched at this point.
Should the secondary survey be performed on scene or should transport be initiated?	Transport should be initiated. A secondary survey should be conducted as soon as possible without delaying transport.

STUDY QUESTIONS

1. You are called to the scene of a possible domestic violence situation and are the first to arrive on scene. As you arrive, you hear a man and woman arguing loudly and a child crying in the background. You hear a loud crash, and the woman cries out. What is your first priority?
   A. Separate the fighting couple to prevent further injury.
   B. Remove the child from the environment.
   C. Assess the scene, noting any potential weapons or other dangers.
   D. Call for law enforcement.

2. Upon entering the house, you note that the female has obvious multiple bruises on her face and a laceration over one cheek. She is holding her right arm, and you note a significant amount of blood flowing from a long gash. This is an example of what type of hemorrhage?
   A. Capillary bleeding
   B. Venous bleeding
   C. Arterial bleeding
   D. Road rash

3. What is the best way to control the bleeding?
   A. Direct pressure
   B. Elevation of the arm above the heart
   C. Tourniquet
   D. Occlusive dressing

4. As your partner begins to control the bleeding, what should you do?
   A. Check the patient's airway and breathing.
   B. Remove the crying child from the scene.
   C. Observe the scene for potential danger.
   D. Remove the abuser from the scene.

5. The patient is wearing long sleeves, and you are having trouble visualizing the wound. What should you do?
   A. Cut the cloth away from the site, avoiding cutting through the slashed area.
   B. Leave the clothing in place. Put gauze over the wound.
   C. Remove the patient's shirt, and place it in a plastic evidence bag.
   D. Cut through the slash on the sleeve, and use the material as a makeshift tourniquet.

ANSWER KEY

Question 1: D
While your first inclination might be to ensure the safety of the victims, you need to ensure your own safety first. Call for law enforcement.

Question 2: B
Venous bleeding leads to a steady flow of dark red blood.

Question 3: A
With venous bleeds, direct pressure is usually sufficient to stop the flow.

Question 4: C
If both providers have all of their attention focused on the patient, the scene can quickly become threatening, and early clues may be missed.

Question 5: A
You should not cut through bullet or knife holes in the clothing of a crime victim. If the clothing is cut, investigators may ask what alterations were made to the clothing, who made them, and why. Any clothing that is removed should be placed in a paper (not plastic) bag and turned over to investigators.

REFERENCES AND FURTHER READING

National Association of Emergency Medical Technicians. *PHTLS: Prehospital Trauma Life Support*. 9th ed. Burlington, MA: Public Safety Group; 2019.

U.S. Department of Health and Human Services. Chemical Hazards Emergency Medical Management: SALT Triage. https://chemm.nlm.nih.gov/salttriage.htm. Updated September 29, 2017. Accessed October 19, 2018.

U.S. Department of Health and Human Services. Chemical Hazards Emergency Medical Management: START Triage. https://chemm.nlm.nih.gov/startadult.htm. Updated September 29, 2017. Accessed October 19, 2018.

SKILL STATION

Primary Survey of a Trauma Patient

1. Assess the scene for safety, and maintain situational awareness.

2. Prior to contact with patient, alert the patient to your presence.

3. Develop a general impression by visually scanning the patient for major (exsanguinating) hemorrhage that requires immediate intervention.

4. Perform a systematic assessment to assess the patient for major (exsanguinating) hemorrhage and wounds.
   A. Assess the upper extremities/shoulder.
   B. Assess the pelvis, and check for instability.
   C. Assess the buttocks and lower extremities.
   D. Assess the neck to identify major bleeds.

5. Perform an assessment of the trauma patient's airway to identify patency, while maintaining cervical spine stabilization.

6. Assess the rate and effectiveness of breathing.
   A. Assess the chest and axilla.
   B. Assess the chest for symmetry and abnormalities.
   C. Assess the patient's back.

7. Check the trauma patient's pulse, and evaluate the patient's circulation status to identify signs of shock.
   A. Assess the abdomen and flanks for injuries, tenderness, or guarding.

8. Assesses the trauma patient's neurologic (disability) status.

9. Expose the patient to address life threats not immediately visible, and take steps to prevent hypothermia.

10. Reassess the effectiveness of prior interventions with each step and at regular intervals.

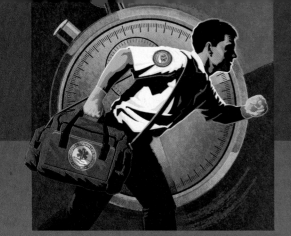

Airway

LESSON OBJECTIVES

· Discuss the potential causes of airway obstruction in a trauma patient.
· Demonstrate the steps of a primary and secondary survey of a trauma patient's airway.
· Choose the most appropriate airway management intervention based on the patient's physical findings.
· Describe the structural differences in the anatomy of adults and children.

Introduction

Two of the most important things you need to know in the prehospital setting are to provide and maintain airway patency and pulmonary ventilation. The failure to adequately ventilate a trauma patient and maintain oxygenation of organs causes additional damage, such as secondary brain injury. Ensuring airway patency and maintaining the patient's oxygenation and supporting ventilation are critical in improving the likelihood of a good outcome.

The respiratory system serves two primary functions:

1. Provides oxygen to the red blood cells
2. Removes carbon dioxide from the body

The inability of the respiratory system to provide oxygen to the cells results in anaerobic metabolism and can quickly lead to death. Failure to eliminate carbon dioxide can lead to coma and acidosis.

PROGRESSIVE CASE STUDY: PART 1

You have been dispatched to the scene where a 20-year-old female was driving a small sport utility vehicle (SUV) on a 4-lane suburban highway at 2100 hours on a clear night (with a temperature of 70°F [21°C]) when she crashed into a tree. She was driving back to her dorm from a house party. She had a slow response to a curve and jerked the steering wheel to the right, running off the road at 50 miles per hour (80 kilometers per hour) and striking a tree in a shallow embankment.

The SUV remained upright with 18-inch (46-cm) intrusion into the engine compartment. The steering wheel air bag failed to deploy, but the side curtain air bags deployed at the time of impact. The patient was wearing her lap and shoulder belt at the time of impact.

Fire and law enforcement personnel are on scene managing traffic and vehicle hazards. Fire personnel are working to pry the driver's side door open upon arrival of emergency medical service (EMS) personnel.

The patient is unconscious, and a fire fighter is maintaining cervical spine stabilization. Bleeding to the nose and a hematoma to the forehead are noted.

Questions:

■ What injuries to the patient do you expect given the scenario?

■ What may be potential vehicle hazards?

■ What may be potential scene hazards?

Anatomy

The respiratory system is comprised of the upper airway and the lower airway, including the lungs. Each part of the respiratory system plays an important role in ensuring gas exchange—the process by which oxygen enters the bloodstream and carbon dioxide is removed.

Upper Airway

The upper airway consists of the nasal cavity and the oral cavity. Air entering the nasal cavity is warmed, humidified, and filtered to remove impurities. Air can also enter the oral cavity, but the warming, humidifying, and filtering functions of the nasal cavity are bypassed. Beyond these cavities is the pharynx, composed of muscle lined with mucous membranes, which runs from the internal nares to the upper end of the esophagus.

The pharynx is divided into three discrete sections:

- The nasopharynx (upper portion)
- The oropharynx (middle portion)
- The hypopharynx (lower portion)

Below the pharynx is the esophagus, which leads to the stomach, and the larynx, which contains the vocal cords and the muscles that make them work, housed in a strong cartilaginous box.

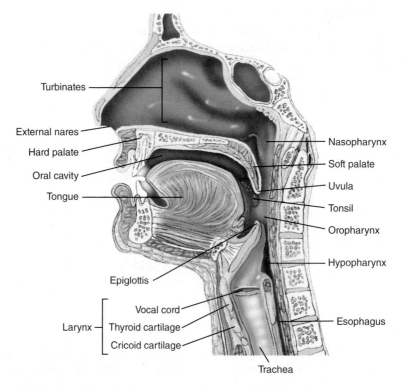

Figure 3-1 Sagittal section through the nasal cavity and pharynx viewed from the medial side.
© National Association of Emergency Medical Technicians.

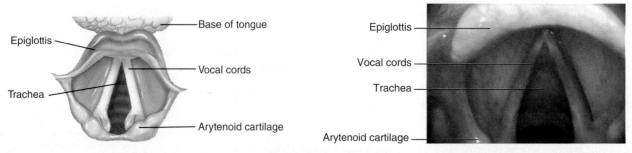

Figure 3-2 Vocal cords viewed from above, showing their relationship to the paired cartilages of the larynx and the epiglottis. Unlike the upper part of the airway, which is all teeth and muscles, the larynx is made up of a thin mucosa and delicate cartilage that won't stand rough treatment.

A: © National Association of Emergency Medical Technicians; **B:** Courtesy of James P. Thomas, M.D., www.voicedoctor.net

Directly above the larynx is a leaf-shaped structure called the epiglottis. Acting as a gate or flapper valve, the epiglottis prevents aspiration of solids and liquids into the trachea during swallowing.

Lower Airway

The lower airway consists of the trachea, its branches, and the lungs. On inspiration, air travels through the upper airway and into the lower airway before reaching the alveoli, where the actual gas exchange occurs. The trachea divides into the right and left main bronchi.

Each of the main bronchi subdivides into several primary bronchi and then into bronchioles (very small bronchial tubes) that terminate at the alveoli, tiny air sacs surrounded by capillaries. The alveoli are the site of gas exchange where the respiratory and circulatory systems meet.

> **FOR MORE INFORMATION**
>
> *Refer to the "Anatomy" section of Chapter 7: Airway and Ventilation.*

Physiology

The airway leads atmospheric air through the nose, mouth, pharynx, trachea, and bronchi to the alveoli. With each breath, the average 150-pound (70-kilogram) adult takes in approximately 500 milliliters (ml) of air.

> **Night of the Living Dead Space**
>
> The airway system holds up to 150 ml of air that never actually reaches the alveoli to participate in the critical gas-exchange process. The space in which this air is held is known as *dead space*.

When atmospheric air reaches the alveoli, oxygen moves from the alveoli, across the alveolar–capillary membrane, and into the red blood cells (RBCs).

The circulatory system then delivers the oxygen-carrying RBCs to the body tissues, where oxygen is used as fuel for metabolism. As oxygen is transferred from inside the alveoli across the cell wall and capillary endothelium, through the plasma, and into the RBCs, carbon dioxide is exchanged in the opposite direction. Carbon dioxide moves from the bloodstream, across the alveolar–capillary membrane, and into the alveoli, where it is eliminated during exhalation.

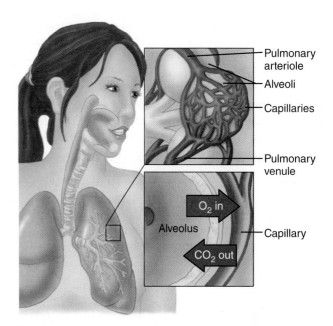

Figure 3-3 Diffusion of oxygen and carbon dioxide across the alveolar–capillary membrane of the alveoli in the lungs.
© Jones & Bartlett Learning.

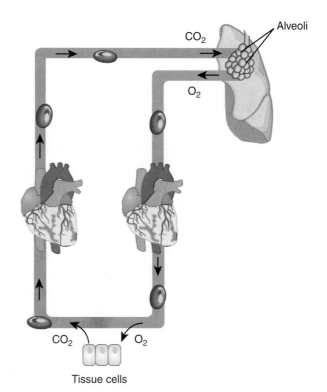

Figure 3-4 Oxygen (O_2) moves into the red blood cells from the alveoli. The O_2 is transferred to the tissue cell on the hemoglobin molecule. After leaving the hemoglobin molecule, the O_2 travels into the tissue cell. Carbon dioxide (CO_2) travels in the reverse direction, but not on the hemoglobin molecule. It travels in the plasma as CO_2.
© National Association of Emergency Medical Technicians.

Assessment of ventilatory function always includes an evaluation of how well a patient is taking in, diffusing, and delivering oxygen to the bloodstream. Without proper intake, anaerobic metabolism begins.

Although the ability to assess tissue oxygenation in prehospital situations is improving rapidly, appropriate ventilatory support for all trauma patients begins by providing supplemental oxygen to help ensure that hypoxia is corrected or averted.

FOR MORE INFORMATION

Refer to the "Physiology" section of Chapter 7: Airway and Ventilation.

Pathophysiology

Trauma can affect the respiratory system's ability to adequately provide oxygen and eliminate carbon dioxide in the following ways:

- Diminished oxygen uptake due to hypoventilation
  - Obstructed airway
  - Hypoventilation due to rib fractures, pneumothorax, or flail chest
  - Diminished oxygen uptake due to lung contusion

Just Breathe

Hypoventilation results from the reduction of minute volume. If left untreated, hypoventilation results in carbon dioxide buildup, acidosis, and eventually death. Management involves improving the patient's ventilatory rate and depth by correcting existing airway problems and assisting ventilation as appropriate.

Hyperventilation can cause vasoconstriction, which can be especially detrimental in the management of the traumatic brain-injured patient, and large tidal volumes can reduce venous return, which can be especially detrimental in shock patients.

The most common cause of upper airway obstruction is the tongue falling backward and obstructing the hypopharynx. This causes airway obstruction along with snoring and abnormal thorax excursions, and in the trauma patient is often further complicated by blood and secretions in the upper airway. This can be corrected by positioning and simple airway maneuvers, such as the trauma jaw thrust or chin lift.

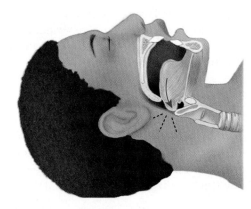

Figure 3-5 The most common cause of upper airway obstruction is the tongue falling backward and obstructing the hypopharynx.
© National Association of Emergency Medical Technicians.

Another common cause is accumulation of secretions, blood, and debris in the hypopharynx when the patient can't clear his or her airway due to decreased level of conciousness (LOC) or extensive trauma.

What's That Sound?

A gurgling respiration is a sure sign that the patient is unable to clear his or her airway and is at risk of aspiration and/or airway obstruction with the very next breath. This condition can be corrected, at least temporarily, by drainage or suction of the upper airway.

The third most common place of upper airway obstruction is the larynx, where obstruction can be caused either by direct trauma to the larynx cartilage

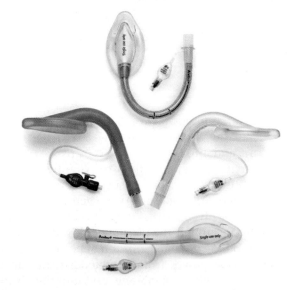

Figure 3-6 Laryngeal mask airway.
Courtesy of Ambu, Inc.

or by inhalation burns with swelling of the mucosa. This condition will manifest with hoarseness and stridor and usually will require an advanced airway endotracheal (ET) tube or surgical airway.

PROGRESSIVE CASE STUDY: PART 2

The patient was thrust into the steering wheel briefly as the SUV struck the tree, due to the steering wheel air bag failing to deploy. There is an abrasion to the patient's throat area just inferior to her mandible, near the area of her thyroid cartilage.

Primary survey shows:

X—Moderate bleeding to nose noted; hematoma to forehead

A—Patient has sonorous and gurgling respirations.

B—Patient has shallow respirations.

C—Patient has a pulse at the radial artery.

D—Patient is unconscious and responsive to painful stimuli; Glasgow Coma Scale (GCS): 7 (E2, V2, M3)

E—Patient remains in the vehicle as the driver's door is stuck.

Questions:

- Is the patient maintaining her airway?
- Do you anticipate any airway issues?
- What additional assessment do you plan to conduct at this point?
- What are the physics of trauma of this crash that concern you regarding the patient's airway?

FOR MORE INFORMATION

Refer to the "Pathophysiology" section of Chapter 7: Airway and Ventilation.

Assessment of the Airway

You need to be able to assess the airway to effectively manage it. A patient who is alert and talking in a normal voice has an open and patent airway. But when the patient's LOC is decreased, it's essential to thoroughly assess the airway prior to moving to other lower priority injuries.

When examining the airway during the primary survey, you need to assess:

- Position of the airway and patient
- Any sounds emanating from the upper airway
- Indirect signs of airway obstruction
- Chest rise

Position of the Airway and Patient

As you make visual contact with the patient, observe the patient's position. Patients in a supine position with a decreased LOC are at risk for airway obstruction from the tongue falling back into the airway.

An unresponsive trauma patient may be placed in the supine position on a backboard for spinal immobilization. Any patient exhibiting signs of decreased LOC will need constant re-examination for airway obstruction and the possible placement of and adjunctive or airway device to ensure an open airway.

Position Matters

Patients with massive facial trauma and active bleeding may need to be maintained in the position in which they are found if they are maintaining their own airway. In some cases, this may mean allowing the patient to sit in an upright position. Placing these patients supine on a backboard may cause obstruction to the airway and possible aspiration of blood.

Airway Evaluation

Noise coming from the upper airway is never a good sign. Upper airway sounds during inspiration are typically due to a partially obstructed airway. The type of sound you hear can give you some clues as to the cause and location of upper airway obstruction.

While snoring, gurgling, and stridor sounds are all critical, stridor can be the hardest to manage. Stridor is a high-pitched whistling sound that can be caused by:

- Direct trauma
- Foreign body
- Swelling of the mucosa, as in inhalation burns

QUICK TIP

Swelling is a challenging situation because it occurs at the narrowest point of the upper airway. You must take steps immediately to alleviate the obstructions and maintain an open airway.

PROGRESSIVE CASE STUDY: PART 3

Vital signs show:

- BP: 154/108 mm Hg
- Heart rate and quality: 70 beats/min at radial
- Ventilation rate: 20 breaths/min, shallow chest rise
- SpO$_2$: 94%/RA
- ETCO$_2$: 40 mm Hg
- Skin condition and temperature: Warm, dry skin
- Temperature: 98.5°F (37°C)
- Pain: 3/10 at throat area

Primary survey reassessment shows:

X—Moderate bleeding to nose noted; hematoma to forehead

A—Open; cervical spine is stabilized

B—Patient continues to present with shallow breathing

C—Patient has a radial pulse.

D—Patient is unconscious and responsive to painful stimuli; GCS 7 (E2, V2, M3); right pupil dilated and unresponsive

E—Patient is extricated and now on backboard away from vehicle.

Questions:

- Is cervical spine stabilization indicated?
- Is airway management indicated?
- What additional assessment can be performed while the patient is still in the vehicle?
- What additional information do you want to know about your patient?
- Based on what we know about the patient, what are our management options?
- Is the patient stable or unstable?
- What is your management plan?
- What is your airway assessment plan?
- How will you determine if the patient has an adequate airway and breathing?
- Does the patient require oxygen?

Limited chest rise can be another sign of airway obstruction. Additional signs, like the use of accessory muscles and the appearance of increased work of breathing during inspiration, should lead to a high index of suspicion of airway compromise.

When a patient is working hard to move air across an obstructed airway, negative pressure builds up in the chest, and you'll see retractions between the ribs and at the jugular notch when muscle and tissues are pulled into the chest. These retractions are especially visible in children. When the airway becomes even more obstructed, "seesaw breathing" or "rocking boat breathing" is likely to occur.

FOR MORE INFORMATION

Refer to the "Assessment of the Airway and Ventilation" section of Chapter 7: Airway and Ventilation.

Management

Airway management is a process. It's critical to assess and properly manage a patient's airway to ensure the patient is able to ventilate.

Management of the airway can be challenging, but in most patients, manual or simple procedures may be sufficient—at least initially. Depending on the situation, these techniques can be applied immediately without any other material than your hands and lead to a better patient outcome than more complex techniques, which require increased time, personnel, and equipment.

To manage the airway, you need to:

- **Assess**—Determine if the airway is open and if the patient can maintain a patent airway.
- **Position**—Many airway issues can be resolved by simple positioning or repositioning to open the airway and keep the tongue from blocking the airway.
- **Suction**—Remove blood and secretions from the airway and clear any debris, broken teeth, etc., before inserting an adjunct or airway device.
  Adjunct
  - Use the appropriate-sized adjunct and use the simplest adjunct needed to maintain the airway.
  - Use a nasopharyngeal or oropharyngeal airway before a supraglottic airway or endotracheal tube.
- **Ventilate**—Ventilate the patient if the patient is not breathing or not effectively ventilating on his or her own.

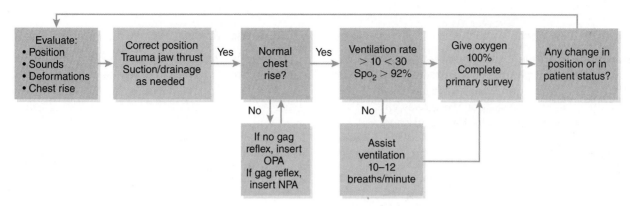

Figure 3-7 Basic airway management algorithm.
© Jones & Bartlett Learning.

- **Oxygenate**—Administer supplemental oxygen as needed, keeping in mind current American Heart Association (AHA) guidelines for oxygen administration to maintain 94% or greater oxygen saturation rate (SpO_2).

> ## QUICK TIP
>
> Always weigh the risk versus the benefit of performing highly invasive complex procedures. These procedures require a high degree of skill proficiency and close oversight by the medical director. They should not be initiated unnecessarily.

Basic Techniques

Airway maintenance skills can be broken into three different levels. The application of these skills should be patient-driven, dependent on the situation and the severity of the patient.

Manual methods of opening the airway are the easiest to use and require no equipment other than your hands. The airway can be maintained with these methods, even if the patient has a gag reflex. There are no contraindications for using manual airway management techniques in a trauma patient. Examples of this type of airway management include the trauma chin lift and the trauma jaw thrust. Positioning and manual clearing of the airway also fall into this category.

The first step in airway management is a quick visual inspection of the oropharyngeal cavity. Foreign material (such as pieces of food) or broken teeth or dentures and blood are swept out of the mouth using a gloved finger or, in the case of blood or vomitus, may be suctioned away.

In unresponsive patients, the tongue becomes flaccid, falling back against the posterior oropharynx and

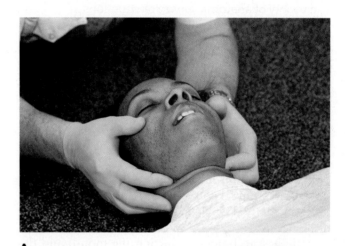

A

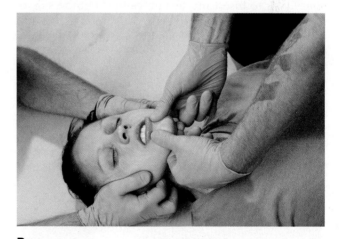

B

Figure 3-8 A. Trauma jaw thrust. **B.** Trauma chin lift.
A: © National Association of Emergency Medical Technicians; **B:** © Jones & Bartlett Learning. Photographed by Darren Stahlman.

blocking the airway. Manual methods to clear this type of obstruction are easy because the tongue is attached to the mandible (jaw) and moves forward with it. Any maneuver that moves the mandible forward will pull the tongue away from the posterior oropharynx.

Trauma Jaw Thrust

In patients with suspected head, neck, or facial trauma, the cervical spine is maintained in a neutral in-line position. The trauma jaw thrust maneuver allows you to open the airway with little or no movement of the head and cervical spine.

Trauma Chin Lift

The trauma chin lift maneuver is used to relieve a variety of anatomic airway obstructions in patients who are breathing spontaneously. The chin and lower incisors are grasped and then lifted to pull the mandible forward. Wear gloves to avoid body fluid contamination.

A trauma patient may require aggressive suctioning of the upper airway. Large amounts of blood and vomit may have already accumulated in the airway. This accumulation may be more than a simple suction unit can quickly clear. The logroll is a quick and efficient method to clear large quantities of vomitus or blood.

The best technique to suction the mouth and the pharynx is to insert the suction catheter in the side of the mouth lateral to the teeth. This approach is less stimulating and can be accomplished even if the patient is clenching his or her teeth.

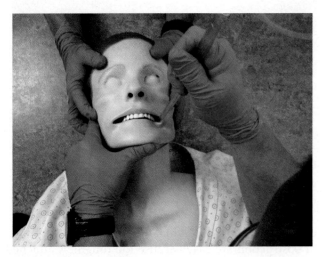

Figure 3-9 Using a rigid suction catheter while maintaining cervical spine alignment.
Photograph provided courtesy of J.C. Pitteloud M.D., Switzerland.

Geriatric Airway

Remember that the geriatric patient's ability to protect his or her airway may be compromised as the result of prior disease.

The most significant complication of suctioning is that suctioning for prolonged periods will produce hypoxemia, which leads to detrimental effects at the tissue level in many organs.

PROGRESSIVE CASE STUDY: PART 4

The patient has blood and secretions in her airway. She remains unconscious and is unable to support her airway.

Questions:

- How do you clear the airway if there are secretions?
- What if the victim begins to vomit?
- Would an oropharyngeal airway (OPA) be useful in this situation?
- What are the contraindications?
- When would you use a nasopharyngeal airway (NPA) in this patient?
- What are the contraindications?
- What do you suspect is going on with the patient?
- How will you manage this patient's airway?
- What is your backup airway plan?
- Would a supraglottic airway work in this situation?

FOR MORE INFORMATION

Refer to the "Management" section of Chapter 7: Airway and Ventilation.

Adult Versus Pediatric Airway Differences

There are several anatomic differences that complicate the care of the injured child. Children have a large occiput and tongue and have an anteriorly positioned airway. Additionally, the smaller the child, the greater the size discrepancy between the cranium and the mid-face, and the large occiput forces passive flexion of the cervical spine.

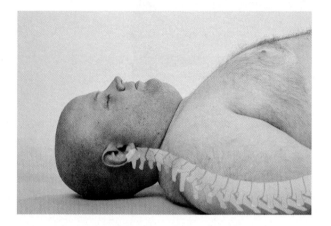

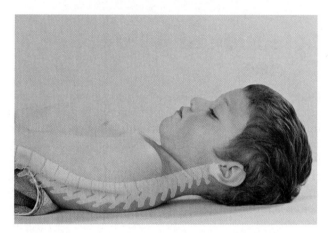

Figure 3-10 Compared to an adult, a child has a larger occiput and less shoulder musculature. When placed on a flat surface, these factors result in flexion of the neck.

A: © Jones & Bartlett Learning. Photographed by Darren Stahlman; **B:** © National Association of Emergency Medical Technicians.

These factors predispose children to a higher risk of anatomic airway obstruction than adults.

You should perform manual stabilization of the cervical spine during airway management and maintain it until a properly sized cervical collar is applied. Placing a pad or blanket of 2 to 3 centimeters thick under an infant's torso can lessen the flexion of the

Protect the Airway!

In the absence of trauma, the pediatric patient's airway is best protected by a slightly superior-anterior position of the midface, known as the sniffing position.

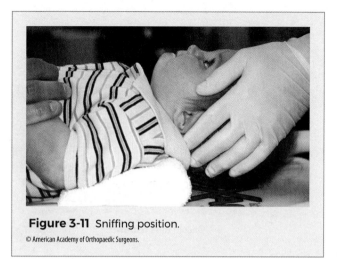

Figure 3-11 Sniffing position.
© American Academy of Orthopaedic Surgeons.

neck and help keep the airway patent. Use bag-mask ventilation with high-flow (at least 15 liters/minute) 100% oxygen when the injured child requires assisted ventilation.

QUICK TIP

Use a properly fitted oxygen mask and the "squeeze-release-release" timing technique. Watch for rise and fall of the chest, and if end-tidal CO$_2$ (ETCO$_2$) monitoring is available, maintain levels between 35 and 40 mm Hg.

If the patient is unconscious, an oropharyngeal airway may be considered, but due to risk of vomiting, do not use it if the patient has an intact gag reflex.

Consider the Epiglottis

When sized properly, the laryngeal mask and King LT airway are supraglottic airways that can be used for airway management in pediatric trauma patients who cannot be ventilated by a simple bag-mask device. In very young children, especially those weighing less than 44 pounds (20 kilograms), these devices can cause iatrogenic upper airway obstruction by causing the relatively larger pediatric epiglottis to fold into the airway.

In comparison to that of the adult, the child's larynx is smaller in size and is slightly more forward and toward the head, making it more difficult to visualize the vocal cords during intubation attempts, so endotracheal intubation should be reserved for those situations in which bag-mask ventilation is ineffective.

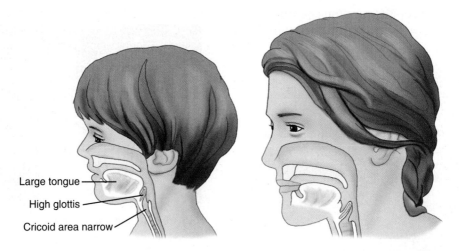

Large tongue
High glottis
Cricoid area narrow

Figure 3-12 Comparison of an adult and child's airway.
© National Association of Emergency Medical Technicians.

CAUTION

Nasotracheal intubation is not recommended in children because it requires a spontaneously breathing patient, involves blind passage around the relatively acute posterior nasopharyngeal angle, and can cause severe bleeding in children. Additionally, in the patient with a basilar skull fracture, it can inadvertently penetrate the cranial vault.

Surgical cricothyroidotomy is usually not indicated in the care of the pediatric trauma patient, though it may be considered in the larger child (usually at the age of 12 years).

PROGRESSIVE CASE STUDY: PART 5

- How will you prepare the patient for intubation?
- How will you prepare to intubate this patient?
- What pharmacologically assisted intubation path will you use?
- What are your assessment points for confirming correct endotracheal tube placement?

FOR MORE INFORMATION

Refer to the "Airway" section of Chapter 14: Pediatric Trauma.

Selection of Adjunctive Device

Once the airway has been opened, airway adjuncts are used in conjunction with positioning to maintain the airway patency. The particular device should be selected based on your level of training and proficiency with a particular device and a risk–benefit analysis. The choice of the airway adjunct should be patient driven, so ask yourself: "What's the best airway for this particular patient in this particular situation?"

Practice Makes Perfect

With complex skills such as intubation or surgical cricothyroidotomy, the more times a skill is performed, the better the chance for a successful outcome. A new paramedic who has performed these procedures only in the classroom setting has less of a chance of intubating a difficult patient successfully compared to an experienced paramedic who has performed these interventions numerous times during his or her career. The more steps there are in a procedure, the more difficult the procedure is to learn and master. These complex skills also lend themselves to a greater probability of failure since greater knowledge is required and more steps are involved in completing the intervention. Generally, the more difficult a procedure is to perform, the greater the risk to the patient of failure or error. With airway procedures, this is particularly true.

There are several types of airway devices that may be selected depending on the needs or potential needs of the patient:

- Simple adjuncts—Devices that lift the tongue from the back of the pharynx only
  - Oropharyngeal airway (OPA)
  - Nasopharyngeal airway (NPA)

  To ventilate requires a mask (usually with bag-mask device)

- Complex airways—Devices that occlude the oral pharynx
  - Supraglottic airways
    - Combitube
    - Laryngeal mask airway (LMA)
    - Laryngeal tubes (LTs) (e.g., King LT)

  Devices that isolate the trachea from the esophagus
  - ET tube
  - Surgical airway

  No mask required to ventilate

Simple Adjuncts

Simple airway management involves the use of adjunctive devices; the technique for inserting the device requires minimal training. The risks associated with these types of airway devices are extremely low compared to the potential benefit of maintaining a patent airway. Examples of these airways include oropharyngeal and nasopharyngeal airways.

Size Matters: The Bariatric Airway

Bariatric patients need more oxygen for their increased metabolic demand, yet their lung capacity doesn't increase with their size. Keep in mind that their normal respiratory rate may be much higher than the average adult.

Complex Airways

Complex airways include airway devices that require significant initial and ongoing training to keep up to date. While complex airways provide greater airway protection compared to basic techniques, their use in the field requires more time and personnel. Devices that fall into this category require multiple pieces of equipment and the possible use of pharmaceuticals as well as multiple steps to insert the airway and, in some cases, direct visualization of the tracheal opening. Surgical airway techniques such as cricothyroidotomy (both needle and surgical) also fall into this category. The risk of failure when using complex airways is high. Examples of these airways include endotracheal tubes and supraglottic airways.

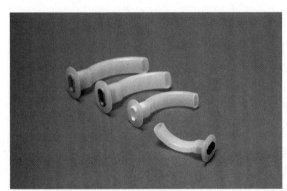

A

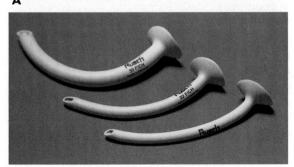

B

Figure 3-13 A. Oropharyngeal airways. **B.** Nasopharyngeal airways.

© Jones & Bartlett Learning. Courtesy of MIEMSS.

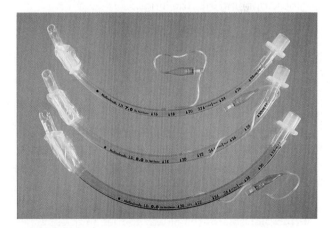

Figure 3-14 Endotracheal tubes.

© Jones & Bartlett Learning.

QUICK TIP

Continuous monitoring of oxygen saturation and ETCO$_2$ is highly recommended when using this group of airways, adding to the complexity of their use.

It's All in the Timing

Transport time may be a factor; an example may be a patient whose airway is being maintained effectively with an OPA and bag-mask with a short transport time to the trauma center. You may elect not to intubate but rather transport while maintaining the airway using simple airway techniques. Providers need to assess the risks versus the benefits when making the decision to perform complex airway procedures.

QUICK TIP

Because techniques and airway devices continue to change, keeping abreast of these changes is important.

Airway Techniques Synopsis

Basic Airway Techniques

Principle: in the normal state the upper airway is open and the esophagus is occluded. Basic life support (BLS) airway maneuvers maintain the upper airway open so that air flows through the glottic opening into the lungs.

Specific skills:

- Positioning
- Suctioning
- Trauma chin lift, trauma jaw thrust
- OPA and NPA

Can be used in a patient with a gag reflex (except OPA)

No airway protection against aspiration

Advanced Airway Techniques

Principle: Isolates the airway so that air goes selectively through the glottic opening into the lungs

Specific skills:

Supraglottic airway devices (LMA, King Airway)

Occludes the esophagus while opening the airway

- Requires an unconscious patient
- Offers only a little protection against aspiration

Endotracheal intubation

Tube goes through the glottic opening into the trachea

- Requires a deeply anesthetized and relaxed patient
- Protects the airway against both aspiration and occlusion through swelling

Surgical airway

Tube goes through the cricothyroid membrane into the trachea

- Because it bypasses the pharynx and the glottis, it can be done in a conscious patient with local anesthesia or no anesthesia at all
- Protects the airway against aspiration

FOR MORE INFORMATION

Refer to the "Selection of Adjunctive Device" section of Chapter 7: Airway and Ventilation.

Continuous Quality Improvement in Intubation

The risk of hypoxia from prolonged intubation attempts for a patient who has a difficult airway needs to be weighed against the need to insert the ET tube in the field.

Factors That Contribute to Difficult Intubation

- Receding chin
- Short neck
- Large tongue
- Small mouth opening
- Cervical immobilization or stiff neck
- Facial trauma
- Bleeding into the airway
- Active vomiting
- Access to the patient
- Obesity

With some literature questioning the effectiveness of prehospital intubation of the trauma patient, the decision to perform endotracheal intubation or to use an alternative device should be made after your assessment identifies the difficulty of the intubation.

It's important that the medical director or his or her designee reviews all out-of-hospital intubations and invasive airway techniques. This is even more important if medications have been used to facilitate the intubation attempt. Specific points include:

- Adherence to protocol and procedures
- Number of attempts
- Confirmation of tube placement and the procedures used for verification
- Outcome and complications
- Proper indications for the use of induction agents if used
- Proper documentation of medication dosage routes and monitoring of the patient during and after intubation
- Vital signs before, during, and after intubation

The mnemonic LEMON has been developed to assist in the assessment of the relative difficulty that will be involved in an intubation. LEMON stands for Look externally, Evaluate the 3-3-2 rule, Mallampati, Obstruction, and Neck mobility.

On the Plus Side . . .

Despite the potential challenges of this procedure, endotracheal intubation remains the preferred method of airway control because it:

- Isolates the airway
- Allows for ventilation with 100% oxygen (fraction of inspired oxygen of 1.0)
- Eliminates the need to maintain an adequate mask-to-face seal
- Significantly decreases the risk of aspiration (vomitus, foreign material, blood)
- Facilitates deep tracheal suctioning
- Prevents gastric distention

FOR MORE INFORMATION

Refer to the "Continuous Quality Improvement in Intubation" section of Chapter 7: Airway and Ventilation.

Pharmacologically Assisted Intubation

Medically assisted intubation of any type requires time. Intubated patients should be sedated for transport according to local protocols. Be aware that sedation may decrease the work of breathing and any "fighting the ventilator" when mechanical ventilation is being used. If sedating the patient, small doses of benzodiazepines should be titrated intravenously.

Table 3-1 Pharmacologically Assisted Intubation

Indications	A patient who requires a secure airway and is difficult to intubate because of uncooperative behavior (as induced by hypoxia, traumatic brain injury, hypotension, or intoxication)
Relative Contraindications	Availability of an alternative airway (e.g., supraglottic)
	Severe facial trauma that would impair or preclude successful intubation
	Neck deformity or swelling that complicates or precludes placement of a surgical airway
	Known allergies to indicated medications
	Medical problems that would preclude use of indicated medications
Absolute Contraindications	Inability to intubate
	Inability to maintain airway with bag-mask device and OPA
Complications	Inability to insert the ET tube in a sedated or paralyzed patient no longer able to protect his or her airway or breathe spontaneously; patients who are medicated and then cannot be intubated require prolonged bag-mask ventilation until the medication wears off.
	Development of hypoxia or hypercarbia during prolonged intubation attempts.
	Aspiration
	Hypotension—virtually all of the medications have the side effect of decreasing blood pressure.

© National Association of Emergency Medical Technicians.

Always exercise caution whenever considering the use of medications for intubation.

Block That Punch

The use of neuromuscular blocking agents may also be considered if the patient is significantly combative, the airway is secured with an ET tube, and prehospital care personnel are qualified in its use. However, patients should *not* receive neuromuscular blocking agents without proper sedation.

FOR MORE INFORMATION

Refer to the "Endotracheal Intubation" section of Chapter 7: Airway and Ventilation.

CRITICAL-THINKING QUESTION

What are the benefits of RSI?

- It allows for the patient to be sedated and maintain muscle tone to prevent the flow of gastric contents up the esophagus and into the airway.

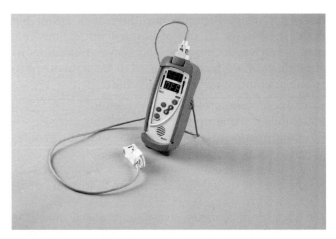

Figure 3-15 A pulse oximeter.
© Jones & Bartlett Learning.

Normal Spo_2 is greater than 94% at sea level. When Spo_2 falls below 90%, oxygen delivery to the tissues is severely compromised.

Rarified Air

At higher altitudes, the acceptable levels of SpO_2 are lower than at sea level. Prehospital care providers should know what Spo_2 levels are acceptable at higher altitudes, if practicing in such settings.

Evaluation

Technological advances have assisted with monitoring the effectiveness of our treatments with such devices as pulse oximetry and capnography. But it's crucial that you always treat your patient and not the monitor. Evaluate the effectiveness of your ventilations, but good chest rise and fall, skin color improvement, mentation improvements, and most of all your patient's vital signs are important indicators.

Pulse Oximetry

Appropriate use of pulse oximetry devices allows early detection of pulmonary compromise or cardiovascular deterioration before physical signs are clear. Pulse oximeters are useful in prehospital applications because of their high reliability, portability, ease of application, and applicability across all age ranges and races.

To ensure accurate pulse oximetry readings, follow these general guidelines:

1. Use the appropriate size and type of sensor.
2. Ensure proper alignment of sensor light.
3. Ensure that sources and photodetectors are clean, dry, and in good repair.
4. Avoid sensor placement on grossly edematous (swollen) sites.
5. Remove any nail polish that may be present.

CRITICAL-THINKING QUESTION

Is pulse oximetry 100% accurate?

- No, it can be affected by multiple situations, particularly when using fingertip probes.

Capnography

Capnography, or end-tidal carbon dioxide ($ETCO_2$) monitoring, has been used in critical care units for many years. Recent advances in technology have allowed smaller, more durable units to be produced for prehospital use. Continuous capnography provides another tool and must be correlated with all other information about a patient.

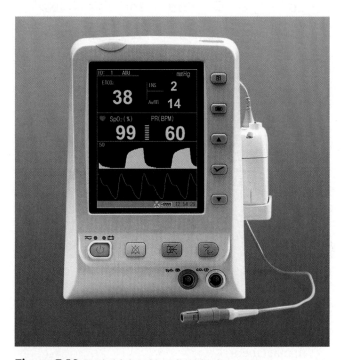

Figure 3-16 End-tidal carbon dioxide detector.

Courtesy of DRE Medical Equipment.

This technique places a sensor directly into the "mainstream" of the exhaled gas. In the patient being ventilated with a bag-mask device, the sensor is placed between the bag-mask device and the ET tube. A normal $ETCO_2$ reading in a critical trauma patient is 30 to 40 mm Hg.

Know When to Monitor

Initial transport decisions are based on clinical findings. For example, it would be inappropriate to take time at the scene to place the patient on monitors if the patient is losing blood. Instead, capnography should be applied en route to the hospital.

Capnography is the gold standard for monitoring proper tube placement and a sudden drop in expired carbon dioxide, as may result either from dislodgement of the ET tube or from decreased perfusion, should prompt a reevaluation of patient status and ET tube position.

QUICK TIP

$ETCO_2$ is the ultimate means to determine that air exchange is taking place. Generally, it's advisable to have a working CO_2 monitor when using an advanced airway.

PROGRESSIVE CASE STUDY: PART 6

During transport, your patient's Spo_2 alarm goes off, displaying a reading of 89%. $ETCO_2$ drops to 35 mm Hg.

Questions:

- How will you monitor the patient after her airway is secured?
- To what type of facility will you transport your patient?

FOR MORE INFORMATION

Refer to the "Evaluation" section of Chapter 7: Airway and Ventilation.

Prolonged Transport

Airway management of a patient prior to and during a prolonged transport requires complex decision making. Interventions to control and secure the airway, especially using complex techniques, depend on a number of factors, including:

- The patient's injuries
- The clinical skills of the provider
- The equipment available
- The distance and transport time to definitive care

Consider the risks and benefits of all the airway options available before making a final airway decision. Both a longer distance of transport and a longer transport time lower the threshold for securing the airway with endotracheal intubation. For transports of 15 to 20 minutes, essential skills, including an oral airway and bag-mask ventilation, may be sufficient. Use of air medical transport also lowers the threshold to perform endotracheal intubation, as a cramped, noisy environment makes ongoing airway assessment and management difficult.

Don't Be a DOPE!

A change in an intubated patient's status requires immediate reassessment.

- Use the DOPE mnemonic.
D—Dislodgement
- Reassess at the ET tube depth from the initial depth during intubation and adjust the ET tube if needed.
O—Obstruction
- Reassess breath sounds and suction the ET tube if needed; if swelling is suspected and occluding the airway, consider a surgical airway.
P—Pneumothorax
- Reassess breath sounds, and perform a needle thoracostomy on the affected side if absent breath sounds are discovered.
E—Equipment
- Check equipment, and swap out if an equipment issue is discovered; if using a ventilator, switch to a bag-mask device and check lung compliance with the bag.

Complete a primary survey.

- Because there has been a change in status, a primary survey should be repeated to address life threats in addition to the DOPE assessment.

Brush Up on Your Math

Prior to the prolonged transport of a patient, you need to calculate potential oxygen needs and be sure sufficient amounts of oxygen are available for the transport. A good rule of thumb is to bring 50% more oxygen than the anticipated need.

Table 3-2 Oxygen Tank Size and Duration

Flow Rate (liter/min)	Tank Size and Duration (in hours)				
	D	E	M	G	H/K
2	2.5	4.4	24.7	38.2	49.7
5	1	1.8	9.9	15.3	19.9
10	0.5	0.9	4.9	7.6	9.9
15	0.3	0.6	3.3	5.1	6.6

Note: This table shows the approximate duration in hours of various sizes of oxygen tanks and flow rates. The numbers are based on the assumption that the oxygen tank is completely full at 2,100 pounds per square inch (psi).

© Jones & Bartlett Learning.

FOR MORE INFORMATION

Refer to the "Prolonged Transport" section of Chapter 7: Airway and Ventilation.

LESSON WRAP-UP

- Trauma airway management can be difficult. Traumatic injuries can result in disruption of airways and structures.

- Know your limitations. If you know that intubation is not your strength, allow someone to do it who is stronger in the skill.

- Start with the basics, then move to advanced management.
  - If a basic adjunct or maneuver manages the airway, stay with it unless an advanced adjunct or technique is needed.

- Practice makes perfect.

- Use a team approach.
  - Have a trauma team plan in place so everyone on the team has a role and time can be saved by tasks being completed simultaneously.

- A failed airway renders all other trauma care fruitless. A patient with no airway will die regardless of any other interventions.

PROGRESSIVE CASE STUDY: SUMMARY

A secondary survey is completed during transport to a level I trauma center. The patient had to have surgery to repair bleeding in the brain. She has since been discharged to a rehabilitation facility and is doing well. The patient travels to colleges to speak against drinking and driving and continues to visit your EMS station to thank you.

Critical Actions:

- Airway assessment to identify potential life threats
- Determination of the best airway to manage the patient
- Reassessment of the airway after management of the airway is completed

PROGRESSIVE CASE STUDY RECAP

Part 1

What injuries to the patient do you expect given the scenario?	Airway obstruction due to trauma
What may be potential vehicle hazards?	Vehicle crashes have inherent hazards to safety that must be assessed and mitigated to ensure scene safety, including: ■ Air bags ■ Bumpers ■ Electrical shorts ■ Fire ■ Fuel leaks ■ Stability
What may be potential scene hazards?	Scene hazards include: ■ Active threats ■ Traffic

Part 2

Is the patient maintaining her airway?	No, she is unconscious with sonorous and gurgling respirations.
Do you anticipate any airway issues?	Possibly, as the patient has not been extricated from the vehicle and is unconscious. Prior to extrication, open airway as best as possible using jaw thrust or modified head tilt chin lift. Suction as necessary and insert oral adjunct.
What additional assessment do you plan to conduct at this point?	Once extricated, repeat the primary survey and check the patient's airway for possible issues, such as broken teeth, lacerations to cheek or tongue, etc.

(continued)

PROGRESSIVE CASE STUDY RECAP (*CONTINUED*)

What are the physics of trauma of this crash that concern you regarding the patient's airway?	Air bag deployment can cause facial injuries and burns, which could impact the patient's airway. However, only the side curtain air bags deployed in this case. The patient struck the steering wheel with her head due to the forces involved with the collision and because she had her seat adjusted to be close to the steering wheel.
Part 3	
Is cervical spine stabilization indicated?	Yes, based on the potential for neck injury to represent a distracting injury that may impede accurate assessment of the potential for a cervical spine injury.
Is airway management indicated?	Yes, due to further assessment and findings supporting traumatic brain injury, hyperventilation should be considered for intracranial pressure to a partial pressure of carbon dioxide in arterial blood target of 30-35 mm Hg.
What additional assessment can be performed while the patient is still in the vehicle?	Observation of depth of breathing, assessment of pulse oximetry, and auscultation of airway and lung sounds.
What additional information do you want to know about your patient?	Unable to assess as she is unconscious.
Based on what we know about the patient, what are our management options?	Further assessment, repeat the primary survey, and treat life threats.
Is the patient stable or unstable?	At this point, the patient is unstable due to signs of increasing cranial pressure.
What is your management plan?	Address airway concerns with an understanding that aggressive ventilation may lead to regurgitation and aspiration. Continue assessment, determine if spinal immobilization is indicated based on neurologic assessment, and package for transport.
What is your airway assessment plan?	Assess the patient's face for stability, examine inside of the patient's mouth for broken teeth or bleeding from cheek/tongue lacerations, examine for possible obstructions.
How will you determine if the patient has an adequate airway and breathing?	Patient is breathing without difficulty, there is adequate symmetrical chest rise, pulse oximetry of 94% or above, and normal lung sounds.
Does the patient require oxygen?	Yes, evidence supports the need for supplemental oxygen. Apneic oxygenation is recommended prior to advanced airway.
Part 4	
How do you clear the airway if there are secretions? What if the victim begins to vomit?	A rigid, large bore catheter would work best. Try to introduce it by the side of the mouth (fewer reflexes, less risk of having the victim biting on the catheter). If she begins to vomit, be ready to logroll her onto her side.
Would an OPA be useful in this situation?	OPA is simple and efficient; check with a tongue blade that the patient has no gag reflex before using.

What are the contraindications for the OPA?	Conscious patients, any patient with a gag reflex.
When would you use an NPA in this patient?	NPA is efficient and well tolerated, even in semi-conscious patients. However, extreme caution should be paid to correct insertion technique (insertion parallel to the palate, not toward the brain). Extreme caution is advised if the patient shows signs of fracture to the basis of the skull.
What are the contraindications for the NPA?	Severe head injury with blood draining from nose, history of fractured nasal bone
What do you suspect is going on with the patient?	The patient has suffered a head injury and is unable to control her airway.
How will you manage this patient's airway?	Elevate the board to facilitate breathing, provide apneic oxygenation while hyperventilating with a bag-mask device, secure airway with supraglottic airway, avoid a tight collar over the neck, and rapidly transport to a trauma facility that is 15 minutes away.
What is your backup airway plan?	Inserting an endotracheal tube might be difficult with this patient. Since the patient is unconscious, consideration must be given to delayed-sequence intubation (DSI)/rapid-sequence intubation (RSI) prior to the intubation. Intubation should only be performed by an experienced provider.
Would a supraglottic airway work in this situation?	Probably not, with controlled hyperventilation an increased risk for aspiration exists. A supraglottic airway is an indirect airway, an endotracheal tube (ET) would be the best option.

Part 5

How will you prepare to intubate this patient?	Gather intubation equipment and ET tubes of at least three sizes, have suction ready, have medications for DSI/RSI ready, and be prepared for your backup plan.
What pharmacologically assisted intubation path will you use?	DSI or RSI could be used, depending on your patient and transport time considerations.
How will you prepare the patient for intubation?	Explain what you are going to do and why, administer DSI/RSI medications, and preoxygenate patient prior to intubation.

What are your assessment points for confirming correct endotracheal tube placement?	■ There are many ways to confirm ET tube placement, some are observational, and some are measured.
	■ Observational
	  1. See the ET tube pass through the vocal cords.
	  2. See misting in the ET tube when the patient exhales.
	  3. See the chest rise during ventilation.
	  4. Auscultate and hear ventilation in both lungs at multiple points.
	  5. Feel bag compliance when ventilating.
	■ Measurable
	  1. Improvement in pulse oximeter readings
	  2. Capnography showing 30 to 40 mm Hg during exhalation
	■ EMS practitioners should assess several observational and measurable assessment points to confirm ET tube placement.

(continued)

PROGRESSIVE CASE STUDY RECAP (*CONTINUED*)

Part 6	
How will you monitor the patient after her airway is secured?	Cardiac monitor with Spo$_2$ and ETCO$_2$, along with the patient's clinical condition with frequent reassessments
To what type of facility will you transport your patient?	A level I trauma center, since the patient has a significant impact with 18-inch (46-cm) intrusion and obvious signs of head injury.

STUDY QUESTIONS

1. You are called to the scene of an explosion and fire at a chemical plant where you find multiple casualties. Triage has begun. Your first patient is a 40-year-old man who was near the source of the explosion. He is unconscious and has extensive injuries. You note gurgling respirations. Why should you use the trauma jaw thrust maneuver first when dealing with a trauma patient?
   A. It's an easy technique that always works to open the airway.
   B. It allows you to open the airway with little or no movement of the head and cervical spine.
   C. Other techniques and interventions don't work as well.
   D. It can relieve a variety of anatomic airway obstructions in patients who are breathing spontaneously.

2. The patient becomes apneic. You suspect he has a cervical injury. Which type of airway should you use?
   A. Supraglottic airway
   B. Blind nasotracheal intubation
   C. Oropharyngeal airway
   D. Surgical airway

3. You have determined that you are going to need to perform orotracheal intubation on this patient. What do you need to do first?
   A. Preoxygenate to maximize oxygen saturation.
   B. Place the patient in a "sniffing" position.
   C. Clear the mouth of any obstructions.
   D. Prepare the patient for immediate transport.

4. You next patient is a fire fighter who was overcome by smoke inhalation during the fire. His trachea is swelling rapidly. What type of airway treatment will he most likely need?
   A. Supraglottic airway
   B. Endotracheal intubation
   C. Trauma chin thrust
   D. Nasopharyngeal airway

5. Why is it important to ensure that the ET tube has been properly placed in the trachea?
   A. Improper placement will cause the patient extreme discomfort.
   B. Oxygen saturation readings will be inaccurate.
   C. Inadvertent esophageal placement of an ET tube may result in profound hypoxia, brain injury, and even death.
   D. You could get sued.

6. Why should you use capnography?
   A. To get accurate readings for hypotension
   B. To assure proper airway placement
   C. To monitor for hyperventilation
   D. To ensure proper placement for needle decompression

7. Why is it important to avoid inadvertent hyperventilation?
   A. It encourages anaerobic metabolism.
   B. More air will leak into the pleural cavity.
   C. It will increase the potential for the patient to go into shock.
   D. It may lead to poor outcomes in traumatic brain-injured patients.

8. Why might it be more difficult to deal with an airway obstruction in a child?
   A. Children are too young to understand what you are trying to do and will likely be uncooperative.
   B. Children have larger heads and tongues so there is a greater potential for airway obstruction.
   C. Children have smaller heads, so there is less room to clear the obstruction.
   D. A child's epiglottis is smaller and stiffer than an adult's.

ANSWER KEY

Question 1: B
Manual maneuvers like the trauma jaw thrust or chin lift are always the first airway maneuver you should take when treating a trauma patient. In patients with suspected head, neck, or facial trauma, the cervical spine is maintained in a neutral in-line position. The trauma jaw thrust maneuver allows you to open the airway with little or no movement of the head and cervical spine.

Question 2: A
The supraglottic airway's greatest advantage is that it can be inserted independent of the patient's position, which may be especially important in trauma patients with high suspicion of cervical injury.

Question 3: A
Before insertion of any invasive airway, the patient is preoxygenated with a high concentration of oxygen using a simple airway adjunct or manual airway procedure.

Question 4: B
Endotracheal intubation is indicated in instances in which there's an inability to maintain a patent airway, decreased LOC, upper airway burns, and/or signs of impending airway obstruction.

Question 5: C
Inadvertent esophageal placement of an ET tube can result in profound hypoxia, so it's important that you confirm proper placement.

Question 6: B
Capnography can monitor proper endotracheal tube placement. It doesn't read hypotension or hyperventilation and is not useful in needle decompression.

Question 7: D
Inadvertent hyperventilation may lead to poor outcomes in traumatic brain-injured patients.

Question 8: B
Children have larger heads and tongues as compared to an adult so there is a greater potential for airway obstruction in a pediatric patient. You must pay special attention to the proper positioning of the pediatric patient to maintain a patent airway.

REFERENCES AND FURTHER READING

Crewdson, K, Lockey, DJ, Røislien, J, Lossius, HM, and Rehn, M. The success of pre-hospital tracheal intubation by different pre-hospital providers: a systematic literature review and meta-analysis. *Critical Care*. 2017; 21(31). https://ccforum.biomedcentral.com/articles/10.1186/s13054-017-1603-7. Accessed November 15, 2018.

Moy, HP. Evidence-based EMS: Endotracheal intubation. *EMS World*. 2015;44(1):30-2, 34. https://www.emsworld.com/article/206057/evidence-based-ems-endotracheal-intubation. Accessed November 15, 2018.

National Association of Emergency Medical Technicians. *PHTLS: Prehospital Trauma Life Support*. 9th ed. Burlington, MA: Public Safety Group; 2019.

SKILL STATIONS

Trauma Jaw Thrust (Single-Provider Technique)

1. In both the trauma jaw thrust and the trauma chin lift, maintain manual neutral in-line stabilization of the head and neck while the mandible is moved anteriorly. This maneuver moves the tongue forward, away from the hypopharynx, and holds the mouth slightly open.

2. From a position above the patient's head, position your hands on either side of the patient's head, fingers pointing caudad.

3. Depending on the size of your hands, the fingers are spread across the face and around the angle of the patient's mandible.

4. Gentle, equal pressure is applied with these digits to move the patient's mandible anteriorly and slightly downward.

Trauma Chin Lift (Two-Provider Technique)

1. From a position above the patient's head, the patient's head and neck are moved into a neutral in-line position, and manual stabilization is maintained by your partner.

2. You are positioned at the patient's side between the patient's shoulders and hips, facing the patient's head.

3. With the hand closest to the patient's feet, grasp the patient's teeth or the lower mandible between your thumb and first two fingers beneath the patient's chin.

4. Pull the patient's chin anteriorly and slightly caudad, elevating the mandible and opening the mouth.

Oropharyngeal Airway Insertion With Use of the Tongue-Jaw-Lift Insertion Method

1. Your partner brings the patient's head and neck into a neutral in-line position and maintains stabilization while opening the patient's airway with a trauma jaw thrust maneuver.

2. Select and measure for a properly sized OPA. The distance from the corner of the patient's mouth to the earlobe is a good estimate for proper size.

3. The patient's airway is opened with the chin lift maneuver. The OPA is turned so that the distal tip enters the mouth with the flanged end pointing toward the top of the patient's head and tilted toward the mouth opening.

4. Insert the OPA into the patient's mouth and rotate it to fit the contours of the patient's anatomy.

5. The OPA is rotated until the inside curve is resting against the tongue and holding it out of the posterior pharynx. The flanges of the OPA should be resting against the outside surface of the patient's teeth.

Oropharyngeal Airway Insertion With Use of the Tongue-Blade Insertion Method

1. Your partner brings the patient's head and neck into a neutral in-line position and maintains stabilization while opening the patient's airway with the trauma jaw thrust maneuver.

2. Select and measure for a properly sized OPA.

3. Pull the patient's mouth open by the chin and place a tongue blade into the patient's mouth to move the tongue forward in place and keep the airway open.

4. Insert the device with the flanged end pointing toward the patient's feet and the distal tip pointing into the patient's mouth, following the curvature of the airway.

5. The OPA is advanced until the flanged end of the OPA rests against the outside surface of the patient's teeth.

Nasopharyngeal Airway Insertion

1. Your partner brings the patient's head and neck into a neutral in-line position and maintains stabilization while opening the patient's airway with the trauma jaw thrust maneuver.

2. Examine the patient's nostrils with a light, and select the one that is the larger and least deviated or obstructed (usually the right nostril).

3. Select the appropriately sized NPA for the patient's nostril, a size slightly smaller in diameter than the size of the nostril opening (frequently the diameter of the patient's little finger).

4. The length of the NPA is also important. The NPA needs to be long enough to supply an air passage between the patient's tongue and the posterior pharynx. The distance from the patient's nose to the earlobe is a good estimate for proper size. (*Note:* The NPA must not be stretched out when measuring this distance.)

5. The distal tip (nonflanged end) of the NPA is lubricated liberally with a water-soluble jelly.

6. The NPA is slowly inserted into the nostril of choice. Insertion should be in an anterior-to-posterior direction along the floor of the nasal cavity. If resistance is met at the posterior end of the nostril, a gentle back-and-forth rotation of the NPA between the fingers will usually aid in passing it beyond the turbinate bones of the nasal cavity without damage. Should the NPA continue to meet with resistance, the NPA should not be forced past the obstruction but rather withdrawn, and the distal tip should be relubricated and inserted into the other nostril.

7. Continue insertion until the flange end of the NPA is next to the anterior nares or until the patient gags. If the patient gags, the NPA is withdrawn slightly.

One-Provider Bag-Mask Device Technique

1. Kneel above the patient's head, providing manual stabilization of the patient's head and neck in a neutral in-line position with your knees.

2. Insert an airway adjunct. Either an OPA or NPA may be used, depending on the patient's injuries.

3. Fit a face mask over the patient's nose and mouth.

4. Hold the face mask in place with firm downward pressure while keeping the patient's airway open. This can be accomplished by placing the third, fourth, and fifth fingers around the mandible and applying slight upward pressure. The thumb and first finger are wrapped around the face mask in the shape of a C near the attachment point where the bag and face mask meet.

5. Squeeze the bag either by hand or by pressing the bag against your body. This action squeezes the air or oxygen from the bag into the patient's lungs.

6. Observe the patient's chest to ensure adequate chest rise with each breath delivered.

7. Observe ventilations to avoid overinflation and appropriate ventilation rate is maintained.

8. Ensure the patient's oxygen saturation is being monitored throughout.

Two-Provider Bag-Mask Ventilation Technique

1. Your partner kneels above the patient's head and maintains manual stabilization of the patient's head and neck in a neutral in-line position.

2. Insert an airway adjunct. Either an OPA or NPA may be used, depending on the patient's injuries.

3. Place the face mask over the patient's nose and mouth.

4. Your partner holds the mask in place with the thumbs on the lateral portion of the mask while pulling the mandible up into the mask. The other fingers provide the manual stabilization and maintain a patent airway.

5. Kneel at the side of the patient and squeeze the bag with both hands to inflate the lungs.

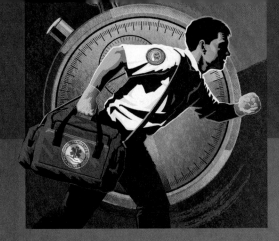

Breathing, Ventilation, and Oxygenation

LESSON OBJECTIVES

- Identify inadequate breathing based on trauma patient assessment.
- Manage life-threatening injuries impairing airway and breathing in a trauma patient.
- Choose the most appropriate airway management intervention through risk versus benefit.
- Choose the most appropriate supplemental oxygen delivery device based on the patient's signs and symptoms.
- Determine when to ventilate and when to oxygenate a trauma patient.
- Monitor the ventilation and perfusion status of a trauma patient using waveform capnography.

Introduction

You already know how important it is to maintain the airway. The next step is ensuring adequate breathing (ventilation and respiration). Several factors can affect the patient's ability to breath, especially when traumatic injuries are involved. These injuries can affect the respiratory system directly (collapsed lung) or indirectly (bruised rib causing pain and decreasing tidal volumes).

The thoracic organs are intimately involved in the maintenance of oxygenation, ventilation, perfusion, and oxygen delivery. Injury to the chest, especially if not promptly recognized and appropriately managed, can lead to significant morbidity.

PROGRESSIVE CASE STUDY: PART 1

You are responding to the practice field of the local high school baseball team. Dispatch informs you that the patient is a 16-year-old male who was struck by a wild pitch during batting practice. He is having difficulty breathing. A level I trauma center is 15 minutes away by ground and a level IV hospital is 5 minutes away by ground.

When you arrive, players direct you to the patient. An athletic trainer is with him and numerous concerned players and coaches are around. The trainer tells you that the patient took a line drive from a fast ball during pitching practice.

The patient is alert and oriented, sitting in a tripod position, and holding the right side of his chest. He appears to be in distress.

Questions:

- What possible injuries would cause a baseball player to have such severe difficulty breathing?
- What part of the patient's anatomy would you expect to be injured?
- What ventilation/oxygenation issues would you expect these injuries to cause?
- Why are these ventilation and/or oxygenation issues being caused?

Physiology

With each breath, air is drawn into the lungs. The movement of air into and out of the alveolus results from changes in intrathoracic pressure generated by the contraction and relaxation of specific muscle groups. The primary muscle of breathing is the diaphragm. Normally, the diaphragm muscle fibers shorten when they receive a stimulus from the brain.

In addition to the diaphragm, the external intercostal muscles help pull the ribs forward and upward. This flattening of the diaphragm, along with the action of the intercostal muscles, is an active movement that creates a negative pressure inside the thoracic cavity and causes atmospheric air to enter the intact pulmonary tree.

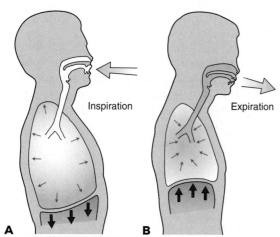

Figure 4-1 When the chest cavity expands during inspiration, the intrathoracic pressure decreases and air goes in the lungs. When the diaphragm relaxes and the chest returns to its resting position, the intrathoracic pressure increases and air is expelled. When the diaphragm is relaxed and the glottis is open, the pressure inside and outside the lungs is equal. **A.** Inspiration. **B.** Expiration.
© National Association of Emergency Medical Technicians.

QUICK TIP

Other muscles attached to the chest wall can also contribute to the creation of negative pressure; these include the sternocleidomastoid and scalene muscles. The use of these secondary muscles will be noticeable as the work of breathing increases in the trauma patient.

In contrast, exhalation is normally a passive process, caused by the relaxation of the diaphragm and chest wall muscles and the elastic recoil of these structures. However, exhalation can become active when air becomes trapped in the lower airways.

You Can't Get Negative Pressure in an Open System

Generating negative pressure during inspiration requires an intact chest wall. In the trauma patient, a wound that creates an open pathway between the outside atmosphere and the thoracic cavity can result in air being pulled in through the open wound rather than into the lungs. Damage to the bony structure of the chest wall can compromise the patient's ability to generate the needed negative pressure required for adequate ventilation.

Assessing ventilatory function should include an evaluation of how well a patient is taking in, diffusing, and delivering oxygen to tissue cells. You need to ensure effective ventilation in your patient. Aggressive assessment and management of any inadequacies in oxygenation and ventilation are critical to a successful outcome.

Oxygenation

The oxygenation process involves the following three phases:

1.   **External respiration** is the transfer of oxygen molecules from air to the blood.

QUICK TIP

The greater the pressure of the gas, the greater the amount of that gas that will be absorbed into the fluid.

2.   **Oxygen delivery** is the result of oxygen transfer from the atmosphere to the red blood cells (RBCs) during ventilation and the

QUICK TIP

The volume of oxygen consumed by the body in 1 minute in order to maintain energy production is known as oxygen consumption and depends upon adequate cardiac output and the delivery of oxygen to the cells by RBCs.

transportation of these RBCs to the tissues via the cardiovascular system.

3. **Internal (cellular) respiration** is the movement, or diffusion, of oxygen from the RBCs into the tissue cells. Metabolism normally occurs through glycolysis and the Krebs cycle to produce energy.

While understanding the specific details of these processes isn't necessary, it's important to have a general understanding of their role in energy production. Because the actual exchange of oxygen between the RBCs and the tissues occurs in the capillaries, anything that interrupts a supply of oxygen will disrupt this cycle.

Adequate oxygenation depends on all three of these phases.

FOR MORE INFORMATION

Refer to the "Physiology" section of Chapter 10: Thoracic Trauma.

PROGRESSIVE CASE STUDY: PART 2

Your primary survey shows the following:

- **X**—None

- **A**—Patent

- **B**—30 breaths/min, limited chest expansion, diminished lung sounds on the right side of the chest, severe difficulty breathing

- **C**—Lips and nail beds are cyanotic.

- **D**—Glasgow Coma Scale (GCS): 15 (E4, V5, M6)

- **E**—Bruising to the right side of the chest; crepitus upon palpation in that area; no chest expansion on the right side of the rib cage

NOTE: *While the steps of the primary survey are taught and displayed in a sequential manner, many of the steps can, and should, be performed simultaneously. This case study will focus on the patient's breathing and how we can improve the patient's breathing.*

Questions:

- What is your general impression?

- What do you notice about the patient's breathing?

- Does the patient need assistance with ventilation or oxygenation? Why?

- What are the indications of life-threatening injuries that will need immediate attention?

- Why is exposing the injured area important for this patient?

- Look at that contusion! If it looks like that on the outside, what does the inside look like?

- Why does the middle of that bruise move in the opposite direction of the rest of the chest?

- What other injuries or complications can a flail segment cause?

- What will you feel when you ask the patient to take a deep breath? What does this tell you?

- When you listen to the patient's lung sounds, what would you hear on the right side?

- What are the treatment priorities of this patient?

- How would you manage the flail segment?

- How would you address the patient's ventilation issues?

- How would you address the patient's oxygenation issues?

- To what type of facility will you transport your patient?

- What assessments and procedures will need to be performed during transport? Why?

Assessment

The first thing to assess in the process of ventilation is chest rise. You should determine if there's adequate and symmetrical chest rise and fall. You should look for three key parameters during the primary survey: ventilation rate, tidal volume, and symmetry of breath sounds.

There are three components to the physical examination: observation, palpation, and auscultation. The assessment should also include a determination of vital signs.

- **Observation**
  - The presence of cyanosis (bluish discoloration of skin, especially around mouth and lips) may be evident in advanced hypoxia.
  - Note the frequency of respirations and whether the patient appears to be having trouble breathing (gasping, contractions of the accessory muscles of respiration in the neck, nasal flaring).
    - Is the trachea in the midline, or deviated to one side or the other?
    - Are the jugular veins distended?
  - Examine the chest for contusions, abrasions, lacerations, and whether the chest wall expands symmetrically with breathing.
    - Does any portion of the chest wall move paradoxically with respiration? (That is, instead of moving out during inspiration, does it collapse inward, and vice versa during exhalation?) Carefully examine any wounds to see if they're bubbling air as the patient breathes in and out.
- **Auscultation**
  - Evaluate the entire chest. Decreased breath sounds on one side compared to the other may indicate pneumothorax or hemothorax on the examined side.
  - Pulmonary contusions may result in abnormal breath sounds (crackles).
- **Palpation**
  - Gently press the chest wall with hands and fingers to assess for the presence of tenderness, crepitus (either bony or subcutaneous emphysema), and bony instability of the chest wall.

> **QUICK TIP**
>
> Repeat determinations of the ventilatory rate during patient reassessment is an important assessment tool in recognizing that a patient is deteriorating. As patients become hypoxic and compromised, an early clue to this change is a gradual increase in the ventilatory rate.

> **QUICK TIP**
>
> Recall that young children are belly breathers (rely heavily on the diaphragm) so when securing them for transport be sure to not restrict their abdomen too tightly.

> **FOR MORE INFORMATION**
>
> *Refer to the "Assessment" section of Chapter 10: Thoracic Trauma.*

Penetrating Injury

With penetrating injuries, objects go through the chest wall, enter the thoracic cavity, and potentially injure the organs within the thorax. When a penetrating wound creates a communication between the chest cavity and the outside atmosphere, air can enter into the pleural space through the wound during inspiration when the pressure inside the chest is lower than the pressure outside the chest. Air accumulates in the pleural space, decreasing the space available for the lung tissue and resulting in partial collapse of the lung. This prevents effective ventilation within the collapsed portion of the lung. Wounds that do not expose the pleural space can also be associated with lung collapse and accumulation of air in the pleural space when the mechanism of injury results in rupture of lung tissue or small airways. In these situations, pneumothorax results when air from the bronchial tree or from the lungs leaks into the pleural space with inspiration.

To make up for the lost ventilation capacity, the respiratory center stimulates more rapid breathing, increasing the work of breathing. The patient may be able to tolerate the increased workload for a time, but if not recognized and treated, the patient is at risk for ventilatory failure, which will be manifested by increasing respiratory distress as the carbon dioxide levels in the blood rise and the oxygen levels fall.

If there is continued entry of air into the chest cavity without any exit, pressure will begin to build within the pleural space, leading to tension pneumothorax.

This condition further interferes with the patient's ability to properly ventilate. It will also impact circulation negatively since venous return to the heart is reduced by the increasing intrathoracic pressure, and shock may ensue.

Lacerated tissues and torn blood vessels bleed. Penetrating wounds to the chest may result in bleeding into the pleural space (hemothorax) from the chest wall muscles, the intercostal vessels, and the lungs.

Penetrating wounds to the major vessels in the chest result in catastrophic bleeding.

Wounds of the lung may also result in bleeding into the lung tissue itself. This blood floods the alveoli, preventing them from filling with air. Alveoli filled with blood can't participate in gas exchange. The more alveoli that are flooded, the more the patient's ventilation and oxygenation may be compromised.

Blunt Force Injury

Blunt force applied to the chest wall is transmitted through the chest wall to the thoracic organs, especially the lungs. This wave of energy can tear lung tissue, which may result in bleeding into the alveoli. In this setting, the injury is called a pulmonary contusion. A pulmonary contusion is essentially a bruise of the lung. It can be made worse by fluid resuscitation. The impact on oxygenation and ventilation is the same as with penetrating injury.

If the force applied to the lung tissue also tears the visceral pleura, air may escape from the lung into the pleural space, creating a pneumothorax and the potential for a tension pneumothorax.

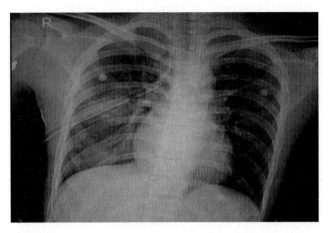

Figure 4-2 An x-ray showing a right pulmonary contusion.
© Kasa1982/Shutterstock.

Blunt force trauma to the chest can also break ribs, which can then lacerate the lung, resulting in pneumothorax as well as hemothorax (both caused by bleeding from the broken ribs and from the torn lung and intercostal muscles). Blunt force injury typically associated with sudden deceleration incidents may cause shearing or rupture of the major blood vessels in the chest, particularly the aorta, leading to catastrophic hemorrhage. Finally, in some cases, blunt force can disrupt the chest wall, leading to instability of the chest wall and compromise of the changes in intrathoracic pressure, leading to impaired ventilation. Remember that ribs are more pliable in pediatric patients, and internal injury is therefore more likely.

PROGRESSIVE CASE STUDY: PART 3

Your secondary survey reveals the following vital signs:

- BP: 118/54 mm Hg
- Heart rate and quality: 128 beats/min, absent radial pulses, weak and thready carotid
- Ventilation rate: 30 breaths/min, shallow and rapid
- SpO_2: 90%/RA
- $ETCO_2$: 48 mm Hg
- Glucose: 120 mg/dl (6.7 mmol/l)
- Skin condition and temperature: Pale, with cyanosis of the lips and nail beds
- Temperature: Warm and dry, 98.7°F (37°C)
- Pain: 7/10 from rib fractures
- GCS: 15 (E4, V5, M6)

Question:

What should be a primary concern?

FOR MORE INFORMATION

Refer to the "Pathophysiology" section of Chapter 10: Thoracic Trauma

Rib Fractures

Rib fractures are present in approximately 10% of all trauma patients. Underlying pulmonary contusion is the most commonly associated injury seen with multiple rib fractures. Compression of the lung may rupture the alveoli and lead to pneumothorax.

Pain relief is a primary goal in the initial management of patients with rib fractures. This may involve reassurance and positioning of the patient's arms using a sling and swath.

It's important to reassure and continuously reassess the patient, keeping in mind the potential for deterioration in ventilation and the development of shock. Encourage the patient to take deep breaths and cough to prevent the collapse of the alveoli (atelectasis) and the potential for pneumonia and other complications.

Administering supplemental oxygen and assisting ventilations may be necessary to ensure adequate oxygenation.

QUICK TIP

Avoid rigid immobilization of the rib cage with tape or straps because these interventions predispose to the development of atelectasis and pneumonia.

Flail Chest

Flail chest occurs when two or more adjacent ribs are fractured in more than one place along their length. The result is a segment of chest wall that is no longer in continuity with the remainder of the chest. When the respiratory muscles contract to raise the ribs up and out and lower the diaphragm, the flail segment paradoxically moves inward in response to the negative pressure being created within the thoracic cavity. Initially, movement may not be noticeable due to muscle spasm and shallow breathing. In this situation, gently palpate for crepitus and auscultate to breath sound changes.

As with a simple rib fracture, the patient will be in pain. The ventilatory rate is elevated, and the patient doesn't take deep breaths because of the pain. The patient may become hypoxic, as shown by pulse oximetry or cyanosis.

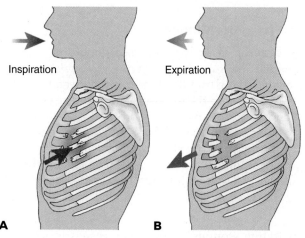

Inspiration   Expiration

A   **B**

Figure 4-3 Paradoxical motion. **A.** If stability of the chest wall has been lost by ribs fractured in two or more places, as intrathoracic pressure decreases during inspiration, the external air pressure forces the chest wall inward. **B.** When intrathoracic pressure increases during expiration, the chest wall is forced outward.

© National Association of Emergency Medical Technicians.

Management of flail chest is directed toward pain relief, ventilatory support, and monitoring for deterioration. It may be necessary to support ventilation with bag-mask device assistance, continuous positive airway pressure (CPAP), or endotracheal intubation and positive-pressure ventilation (PPV) (particularly with prolonged transport times) for patients having difficulty maintaining adequate oxygenation. CPAP and PPV will exacerbate any pneumothorax, converting it to a tension pneumothorax quickly.

Open Pneumothorax

Open pneumothorax involves air entering the pleural space, causing the lung to collapse. This occurs from

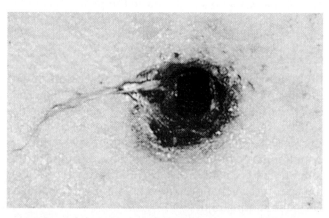

Figure 4-4 A gunshot or stab wound to the chest produces a hole in the chest wall through which air can flow both into and out of the pleural cavity.

Courtesy Norman McSwain, MD, FACS, NREMT-P.

penetrating trauma allowing air from the environment to enter into the chest wall. When the patient attempts to inhale, air crosses the open wound and enters the pleural space because of the negative pressure created in the thoracic cavity as the muscles of respiration contract. In larger wounds, there may be free flow of air in and out of the pleural space with the different phases of respiration.

Assessment of the patient with open pneumothorax usually reveals obvious respiratory distress. The patient will typically be anxious and tachypneic (breathing rapidly). Initial management of an open pneumothorax involves sealing the defect in the chest wall and administering supplemental oxygen.

> **QUICK TIP**
>
> The best way to prevent airflow through the wound into the pleural cavity is by applying an occlusive dressing; using a commercial product such as the Halo, Asherman, or Bolin chest seals; or using improvised methods, such as application of aluminum foil or plastic wrap (unlike plain gauze, these materials do not allow airflow through them). Petroleum gauze is a viable option if a commercial device is not available.

If these measures fail to support the patient adequately, endotracheal intubation and positive-pressure ventilation may be necessary. If you use positive pressure and a dressing to seal the open wound, you need to monitor the patient carefully for the development of tension pneumothorax. If signs of increasing respiratory distress develop, vent or remove the dressing over the wound to allow for decompression of any accumulating tension. If this is ineffective, consider needle decompression.

Tension Pneumothorax

Tension pneumothorax is a life-threatening emergency. As air continues to enter the pleural space without any exit or release, intrathoracic pressure builds up. As intrathoracic pressure rises, ventilatory compromise increases and venous return to the heart decreases. The decreasing cardiac output coupled with worsening gas exchange results in profound shock. The findings during assessment depend on how much pressure has accumulated in the pleural space.

Initially, patients will be apprehensive and uncomfortable. They'll generally complain of chest pain and difficulty breathing. As the tension pneumothorax worsens, they'll exhibit increasing agitation, tachypnea, and respiratory distress. In severe cases, cyanosis, apnea, and cardiac arrest may occur.

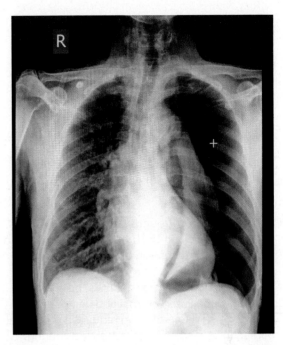

Figure 4-5 An x-ray showing a left tension pneumothorax.
© Noppadon Seesuwan/Shutterstock.

> **Signs of Tension Pneumothorax**
>
> Although the following signs are frequently discussed with a tension pneumothorax, many may not be present or are difficult to identify in the field.
>
> **Observation**
>
> - *Cyanosis* may be difficult to see in the field. Poor lighting, variation in skin color, and dirt and blood associated with trauma often render this sign unreliable.
> - *Distended neck veins* are described as a classic sign of tension pneumothorax. However, since a patient with a tension pneumothorax may also have lost a considerable amount of blood, distended neck veins may not be prominent.
>
> **Palpation**
>
> - *Subcutaneous emphysema* is a common finding. As the pressure builds up within the chest cavity, air will begin to dissect through the tissues of the chest wall. Because tension pneumothorax involves significantly elevated intrathoracic pressure, the subcutaneous emphysema can often be palpated across the entire chest wall and neck and sometimes can involve the abdominal wall and face as well.

- *Tracheal deviation* is usually a late sign. Even when it is present, it can be difficult to diagnose by physical examination. In the neck, the trachea is bound to the cervical spine by fascial and other supporting structures; thus, the deviation of the trachea is more of an intrathoracic phenomenon, although deviation may be palpated in the jugular notch if it is severe. Tracheal deviation is not often noted in the prehospital environment.

Auscultation

- *Decreased breath sounds on the injured side.* The most helpful part of the physical examination is checking for decreased breath sounds on the side of the injury. However, to use this sign, the prehospital care provider must be able to distinguish between normal and decreased sounds. Such differentiation requires a great deal of practice. Listening to breath sounds during every patient contact will help. Most of the time, however, breath sounds are downright absent.

The management priority involves decompressing the tension pneumothorax. You should perform decompression when the following three findings are present:

1. Worsening respiratory distress or difficulty ventilating with a bag-mask device
2. Unilateral decreased or absent breath sounds
3. Decompensated shock (systolic blood pressure less than 90 mm Hg with a narrowed pulse pressure)

Chest decompression is performed with a large-bore (10- to 16-gauge) IV catheter at least 3.5 inches long. The needle and catheter should be advanced until you encounter a rush of air, but not beyond that point. Once you've decompressed the affected side, you'll need to monitor the patient carefully.

Should I Take the Dressing Off?

In the patient with an open pneumothorax, if an occluding dressing has been applied, it should be briefly opened or removed. This should allow the tension pneumothorax to decompress through the wound with a rush of air. This procedure may need to be repeated periodically during transport if symptoms of tension pneumothorax recur. If removing the dressing for several seconds is ineffective or if there is no open wound, an advanced life support (ALS) provider may proceed with a needle thoracostomy.

Hemothorax

Hemothorax occurs when blood enters the pleural space. Because this space can accommodate a large volume of fluid (2,500 to 3,000 ml), hemothorax can represent a source of significant blood loss. In fact, the loss of circulating blood volume from bleeding into the pleural space represents a greater physiologic insult to the patient with chest injury than the collapse of the lung that the hemothorax produces.

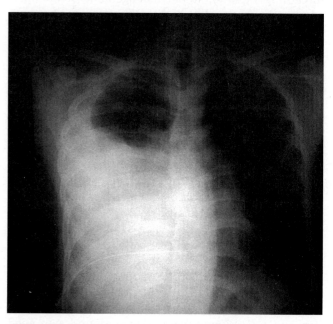

Figure 4-6 An x-ray showing a right hemothorax.
© Medicshots/Alamy Stock Photo.

Assessment usually shows a patient in some distress, depending on the amount of blood lost into the chest and the resultant compression of the lung on the involved side. Chest pain and shortness of breath are prominent features, generally with signs of significant shock. Breath sounds on the side of the injury are diminished or absent.

Pneumothorax may be present in conjunction with hemothorax, increasing the likelihood for cardiorespiratory compromise. Management includes constant observation to detect physiologic deterioration while providing appropriate support. Administer high-concentration oxygen and support ventilation if necessary with bag-mask device or endotracheal intubation, if available and indicated.

FOR MORE INFORMATION

Refer to the "Assessment of Specific Injuries" section of Chapter 10: Thoracic Trauma.

Ventilatory Devices

All trauma patients receive appropriate ventilatory support with supplemental oxygen to ensure that hypoxia is corrected or averted entirely. In deciding which method or equipment to use, consider the following devices and their respective oxygen concentrations.

Bag-Mask Device

The bag-mask device consists of a self-inflating bag and a nonrebreathing device; it can be used with simple (oropharyngeal, nasopharyngeal) airway adjuncts or complex (endotracheal, nasotracheal) airway devices. Adult bag-mask devices have a volume of 1,600 ml and can deliver an oxygen concentration of 90% to 100%. Some models also have a built-in colorimetric carbon dioxide detector. While not "very glamourous," the bag-mask device is the number one tool of most prehospital providers and can be lifesaving if used properly.

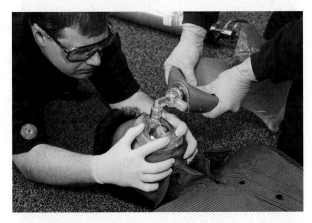

Figure 4-7 Bag-mask device.
© National Association of Emergency Medical Technicians.

> QUICK TIP
>
> A single provider attempting to ventilate with a bag-mask device may create poor tidal volumes secondary to the inability both to create a tight face seal and to squeeze the bag adequately. Ongoing practice is necessary to ensure that the technique is effective and that the trauma patient receives adequate ventilatory support.

Positive-Pressure Ventilators

Positive-pressure volume ventilators during prolonged transport have long been used in the aeromedical environment. However, more ground units are now adopting the use of mechanical ventilation as a means of controlling rate, depth, and minute volume in trauma patients. Only volume ventilators with appropriate alarms and pressure control/relief should be used. These ventilators don't need to be as sophisticated as the ones used in the hospital and only have a few simple modes of ventilation.

- **Assist Control (A/C) Ventilation** is probably the most widely used mode of ventilation in prehospital transport from the scene to the ED. The A/C setting delivers ventilations at a preset rate and tidal volume. If patients initiate a breath on their own, an additional ventilation of the full tidal volume is delivered, which may lead to breath-stacking and overinflation of the lungs.
- **Intermittent Mandatory Ventilation (IMV)** delivers a set rate and tidal volume to patients. If patients initiate a breath, only the amount that they actually inhale on their own will be delivered.
- **Positive End-Expiratory Pressure (PEEP)** provides an elevated level of pressure at the end of expiration, keeping the alveolar sacs and small airways open and filled with air for a longer time. This intervention provides greater oxygenation.

> QUICK TIP
>
> By increasing the end-expiratory pressure and the overall intrathoracic pressure, PEEP may decrease blood return to the heart. In hemodynamically unstable patients, PEEP may further decrease blood pressure. PEEP should also be avoided in patients with traumatic brain injuries since the increase in thoracic pressure can cause an elevation in intracranial pressure.

> FOR MORE INFORMATION
>
> *Refer to the "Ventilatory Devices" section of Chapter 7: Airway and Ventilation.*

Evaluation of Ventilation and Perfusion

Capnography

Capnography, or end-tidal carbon dioxide ($ETCO_2$) monitoring, has been used in critical care units for many years. Recent advances in technology have allowed smaller, more durable units to be produced for prehospital use.

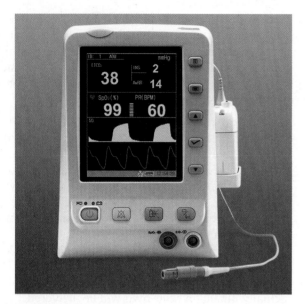

Figure 4-8 Capnography.
Courtesy of DRE Medical Equipment.

Most critical care units in the hospital setting use the mainstream technique. This technique places a sensor directly into the "mainstream" of the exhaled gas. In the patient being ventilated with a bag-mask device, the sensor is placed between the bag-mask device and the endotracheal (ET) tube. An expected ETCO$_2$ reading in a critical trauma patient is 30 to 40 mm Hg. This number represents the partial pressure of carbon dioxide (CO$_2$) detected at the end of exhalation. The graph (waveform) shows how much CO$_2$ is present in each phase of the respiratory cycle.

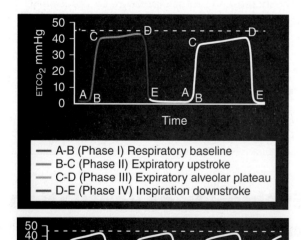

— A-B (Phase I) Respiratory baseline
— B-C (Phase II) Expiratory upstroke
— C-D (Phase III) Expiratory alveolar plateau
— D-E (Phase IV) Inspiration downstroke

Figure 4-9 Capnography. Normal end-tidal wave for capnography. The left side shows that air is moving easily and quickly out of the lungs. The right side shows that air is moving quickly and easily into the lungs. The top shows how easily the alveoli empty.
© Jones & Bartlett Learning.

These next waveforms each show how the capnography waveform is affected by different patient conditions. The first shows a patient with return of spontaneous circulation (ROSC) after cardiac arrest. The second waveform shows a patient trending down in shock. The third waveform indicates a patient experiencing hypoxia due to asthma. Each condition has a different effect on how easily air can move into and out of the lungs and alveoli.

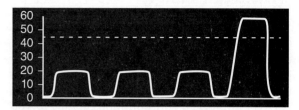

Figure 4-10 Capnography waveform indicating ROSC after cardiac arrest.
© Jones & Bartlett Learning.

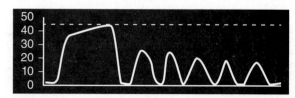

Figure 4-11 Capnography waveform trending down in shock.
© Jones & Bartlett Learning.

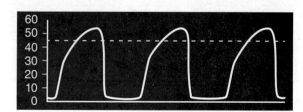

Figure 4-12 Capnography waveform indicating hypoxia due to asthma.
© Jones & Bartlett Learning.

Continuous capnography provides another tool in the prehospital management of a trauma patient and must be correlated with all other information about a patient. Understanding these waveforms will give you an early insight as to what is happening with your patient.

Capnography is the gold standard for monitoring proper tube placement, and a sudden drop in expired

> ### QUICK TIP
>
> Initial transport decisions should be based on physical and environmental conditions. For example, it would be inappropriate to take time at the scene to place the patient on monitors if the patient is losing blood. Capnography should be applied en route to the hospital in such a situation.

carbon dioxide should prompt a reevaluation of patient status and ET tube position. $ETCO_2$ is the ultimate means to confirm that air exchange with the lung is taking place.

> ## QUICK TIP
>
> As a general rule, it's advisable to have a working CO_2 monitor when using an advanced airway.

> ## FOR MORE INFORMATION
>
> *Refer to the "Ventilatory Devices" section of Chapter 7: Airway and Ventilation.*

Prolonged Transport

Priorities for managing patients with known or suspected thoracic injuries during prolonged transport include managing the airway, supporting ventilation and oxygenation, controlling hemorrhage, and providing appropriate volume resuscitation. When faced with a prolonged transport, you may have a lower threshold for securing the airway with endotracheal intubation.

Provide oxygen to maintain oxygen saturation at 94% or greater and assist ventilations as necessary. Pulmonary contusions worsen over time, and the use of CPAP, positive end-expiratory pressure (PEEP) with a transport ventilator, or PEEP valves with bag-mask device may facilitate oxygenation.

Any patient with significant thoracic trauma may have or develop a tension pneumothorax, and ongoing assessment should look for the hallmark signs. In the presence of decreased or absent breath sounds, worsening respiratory distress, difficulty squeezing the bag-mask device, increasing peak inspiratory pressures in patients on a ventilator, and hypotension, you should perform pleural decompression.

> ## QUICK TIP
>
> A tube thoracostomy (insertion of a chest tube) may be performed by authorized personnel, typically air medical flight crews, if the patient requires needle decompression or is found to have an open pneumothorax.

> ## PROGRESSIVE CASE STUDY: SUMMARY
>
> A secondary survey was completed en route. The patient was transported to a level I trauma center where he was treated as an adult for a flail segment and large pulmonary contusion. He was intubated and admitted to the intensive care unit (ICU). He recovered after a short stay and returned to the baseball team.
>
> ### Critical Actions:
>
> - Airway and breathing assessment to identify and manage potential life threats
> - Determining the best method to manage breathing difficulty in this patient and prevent further decline
> - Reassessment of the airway after management of the airway is completed to ensure improvement of the patient's condition

> ## FOR MORE INFORMATION
>
> *Refer to the "Prolonged Transport" sections of Chapter 7: Airway and Ventilation and Chapter 10: Thoracic Trauma.*

LESSON WRAP-UP

- Ventilation is the ability of the body to breathe; oxygenation is the ability of the body to exchange gases.
- Methods in which a patient can be oxygenated include:
  - Nasal cannula
  - Nonrebreathing mask
  - Bag-mask device
  - High-flow nasal cannula
- Airway adjuncts used to increase the ability to ventilate a patient include:
  - Nasopharyngeal airway (NPA)
  - Oropharyngeal airway (OPA)
  - Supraglottic airway
  - Endotracheal tube
  - Needle cricothyrotomy
  - Surgical cricothyrotomy
  - Needle thoracostomy
- Tools used to assess the patient's ventilation and oxygenation status include:
  - Continuous waveform capnography
  - Pulse oximetry (SpO_2)
  - The prehospital provider's skill of observation and auscultation

PROGRESSIVE CASE STUDY RECAP

Part 1

What possible injuries would cause a baseball player to have such severe difficulty breathing?	■ Broken ribs ■ Flail section ■ Pulmonary contusion ■ Pneumothorax ■ Tension pneumothorax ■ Diaphragmatic rupture ■ Sternal fracture ■ Cardiac contusion
What part of the patient's anatomy would you expect to be injured?	■ Ribs ■ Lungs ■ Diaphragm ■ Sternum
What ventilation/oxygenation issues would you expect these injuries to cause?	■ Pain from broken ribs ■ Pain and lung expansion issues from flail section ■ Blood filling the alveoli from a pulmonary contusion restricting oxygen and carbon dioxide exchange ■ Pain and lack of ability to exchange oxygen and carbon dioxide due to collapsed lung and/or buildup of air outside of the lung that causes pressure on the deflated lung and the heart ■ Rupture or laceration of the muscle (diaphragm) that allows chest movement to make respirations possible
Why are these ventilation and/or oxygenation issues being caused?	■ Possible musculoskeletal injuries will cause the patient to have difficulty being able to breath (broken ribs, collapsed lung, lacerated diaphragm), which will necessitate the support of the patient's ventilations (ability to take a breath). ■ The side effects of these injuries—blood in the alveoli, contusions to the lungs, pneumothorax/tension pneumothorax, subcutaneous emphysema—will cause the exchange of oxygen and carbon dioxide to be disrupted, thus causing a ventilation/oxygenation issue.

Part 2

What is your general impression?	The patient is alert, holding himself up in a seated tripod position, and he can speak in short bursts. He is alert with a patent airway and is breathing/ventilating well enough to hold himself up and to speak in an oriented manner.
What do you notice about the patient's breathing?	The patient has quick, shallow respirations, and only able to speak in quick bursts.
Does the patient need assistance with ventilation or oxygenation? Why?	Yes. Even prior to exposing or palpating the patient's chest wall, the rapid, shallow nature of the patient's respirations can't be sustained for long. The story from the trainer stating that the patient took a line drive from a fast ball during pitching practice should give you the suspicion of broken ribs and pulmonary contusion. If the patient's alveoli are filling with blood, he won't be able to efficiently exchange oxygen and carbon dioxide. This patient will need supplemental oxygen to provide additional available oxygen for exchange and possibly respiratory support with positive pressure ventilations.

What are the indications of life-threatening injuries that will need immediate attention?	Broken ribs and flail segments can cause pneumothorax, which will require immediate treatment.
Why is exposing the injured area important for this patient?	Exposing this patient's chest will show you the extent of injury and will increase your suspicions of other injuries that might be affecting his ventilation/ oxygenation status.
Look at that contusion! If it looks like that on the outside, what does the inside look like?	Contusions on the outside of the body should give you a high suspicion that there are contusions of equal or greater size on the inside of the body.
Why does the middle of that bruise move in the opposite direction of the rest of the chest?	The center of that contusion has paradoxical movement.
What other injuries or complications can a flail segment cause?	A flail segment can cause bleeding due to the breaks in the rib cage, pulmonary contusion from ragged bone edges, or pneumothorax or tension pneumothorax.
What will you feel when you ask the patient to take a deep breath? What does this tell you?	The patient complains it's painful to inhale. You may or may not feel paradoxical motion, so it will not likely be visible. Initially, the intercostal muscles will spasm and stabilize the flail segment. As these muscles fatigue over time, the paradoxical motion becomes increasingly evident. The patient will have tenderness and potentially bony crepitus over the injured segment.
When you listen to the patient's lung sounds, what would you hear on the right side?	Any patient with respiratory distress and diminished breath sounds should be assumed to have a pneumothorax. A silent chest usually means no air is moving at all.
What are the treatment priorities of this patient?	Support the patient's ventilation and oxygenation status. The patient may have two mechanisms to compromise ventilation and gas exchange: the flail segment and the underlying pulmonary contusion. The pulmonary contusion prevents gas exchange in the contused portion of the lung because of alveolar flooding with blood. Support ventilation with bag-mask device assistance or continuous positive airway pressure. Continuous assessment of this patient is essential.
How would you manage the flail segment?	Focus on pain management, balancing that without decreasing the ventilatory rate or effort. Oxygen therapy may possibly benefit this patient. Monitor him for deterioration.
How would you address the patient's ventilation issues?	Provide pain relief to alleviate the patient's ability to breathe adequately.
How would you address the patient's oxygenation issues?	Supplemental oxygen and constant monitoring of SpO_2 and $ETCO_2$ will ensure that you catch a deteriorating patient early.

(continued)

PROGRESSIVE CASE STUDY RECAP (CONTINUED)

To what type of facility will you transport your patient?	This patient should be transported to a level I trauma center.
What assessments and procedures will need to be performed during transport? Why?	The secondary survey and IVs should be performed during transport.
Part 3	
What should be a primary concern?	As you move toward positive pressure ventilatory support, keep in mind that this type of ventilation can cause a pneumothorax. In such a case, you would need to perform needle decompression.

STUDY QUESTIONS

1. You're responding to a convenience store where a 36-year-old man was stabbed. You find the patient sitting upright leaning forward. He tries to tell you what happened but has to stop after every five to six words to catch his breath. You notice a gaping laceration approximately 2 inches long in his upper right chest with a small amount of blood-tinged, "bubbling" fluid. The patient is diaphoretic and has a rapid radial pulse. You note decreased breath sounds on the right side with auscultation. No other abnormal physical findings are noted. What's your general impression?
   A. Simple pneumothorax
   B. Open pneumothorax
   C. Hemothorax
   D. Hemopneumothorax

2. What is the first intervention you should take?
   A. Stop the bleeding.
   B. Administer supplemental oxygen.
   C. Apply an occlusive dressing.
   D. Obtain IV access.

3. Unfortunately, you don't have a vented chest seal in your kit. Which of the following should you use instead?
   A. Grab a piece of foil off a shelf, fold it into a square, and tape it on three sides.
   B. Use petroleum gauze to keep the air out.
   C. Leave it open to allow for gas exchange.
   D. Use your gloved hand. That way you can release pressure if you need to.

4. The patient's breathing is starting to get worse. What should you do?
   A. Put pressure around the edges of the dressing to prevent airflow into the wound.
   B. Remove the dressing immediately, and use A/C ventilation.
   C. Leave the dressing alone, and use intermittent mandatory ventilation.
   D. Remove the dressing for a few seconds, and assist ventilations with a bag-mask device.

5. Things aren't going well. The patient's breathing is not improving. In fact, breath sounds continue to diminish on the side of the injury. What is most likely happening?
   A. Bleeding into the alveolar air spaces is resulting in pulmonary contusion.
   B. Air is trapped in the pleural space, increasing intrathoracic pressure. This indicates a tension pneumothorax.
   C. Blood is trapped in the pleural space; he's got a hemothorax.
   D. The stab wound has broken ribs leading to flail chest.

6. The patient has become hypoxic and is not responding to your attempts at oxygenation. His systolic pressure has dropped to 85 mm Hg. What's your next step?
   A. Remove the dressing.
   B. Intubate.
   C. Perform needle thoracostomy.
   D. Perform tube thoracostomy.

ANSWER KEY

Question 1: B
The location of the wound, bubbling fluid, and decreased breath sounds indicate an open pneumothorax.

Question 2: C
The first step is to apply an occlusive dressing to prevent airflow into the pleural cavity.

Question 3: A
If you don't have a vented chest seal, PHTLS recommends using foil or plastic taped on three sides. If these aren't available, an unvented chest seal or a material such as petroleum gauze that prevents ingress and egress of air can be used.

Question 4: D
If the patient develops tachycardia, tachypnea, or other indications of respiratory distress, remove the dressing for a few seconds, and assist ventilations as necessary.

Question 5: B
Because it's an open wound, the most likely suspicion is that air trapped in the pleural space is increasing intrathoracic pressure. This indicates a tension pneumothorax.

Question 6: B
Use positive-pressure ventilatory assistance if the patient is hypoxic and fails to respond to supplemental oxygen.

REFERENCES AND FURTHER READING

National Association of Emergency Medical Technicians. *PHTLS: Prehospital Trauma Life Support.* 9th ed. Burlington, MA: Public Safety Group; 2019.

SKILL STATION

Needle Decompression

1. Don personal protective equipment.
2. Identify the fifth intercostal space along the anterior axillary line on the affected side.
3. Clean the site with an antimicrobial solution (alcohol or betadine).
4. Insert a large-bore (10- to 14-gauge) IV needle that is at least 3.5 inches (8 cm) in length. For lateral decompression, insert the needle in the fifth intercostal space along the anterior axillary line.
5. As the needle enters the pleural space, a "pop" is felt, followed by a possible hiss of air. Ensure that the needle is advanced all the way to the hub.
6. Remove the needle, leaving the catheter secured in place.
7. If tension pneumothorax recurs (as noted by return of respiratory distress), repeat the needle decompression on the injured side.
8. Stabilize the catheter hub to the chest wall with adhesive tape.
9. Listen for increased breath sounds, or observe decreased respiratory distress.
10. Remove gloves, and dispose of them appropriately.

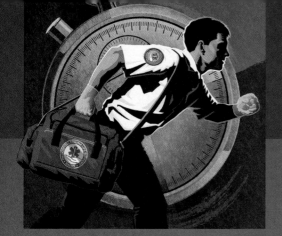

Circulation

LESSON OBJECTIVES
· Describe shock pathophysiology.
· Recognize the clinical signs of shock.
· Explain basic shock treatment.
· Identify the modalities of fluid replacement.
· Explain the role of blood component replacement in the management of hemorrhagic shock.
· Describe special considerations in shock management (age, athletes, hypothermia, medications, pacemakers, and pregnancy).

Introduction

A major complication of disruption of the normal physiology of life is known as *shock*. Shock results from a lack of oxygen to the tissues. It is a highly time-sensitive

issue because our bodies have no real oxygen reserves. We have fat stores for 30 days and glucose stores for 1 day, but we have only enough oxygen reserves for about 5 minutes. If oxygen supply to the tissues is interrupted, organ damage sets in within minutes and, at

PROGRESSIVE CASE STUDY: PART 1

Presentation/Dispatch

You have been dispatched to the scene of a 40-year-old male who has been in a motor vehicle collision. His motorcycle went out of control while trying to pass a car. You find the patient lying on the ground with blood noted around him.

The scene size-up shows that the motorcycle is lying on the side of the street, and the traffic has been stopped by law enforcement. The general impression shows the patient is lying in a pool of blood beside his bike. The bike is not deformed. The primary survey shows:

- **X:** Profuse bleeding from anterior neck wound
- **A:** Tenuous, with sonorous respirations
- **B:** Fast, shallow chest rise
- **C:** Rapid, thready radial pulse
- **D:** Unconscious, moves all extremities to painful stimulus
- **E:** Lying on ground next to his bike

Questions:

- Is the patient in shock?
- What is the definition of shock?
- Why is shock so time sensitive?
- What is special about oxygen transport in the blood?
- Is loss of red blood cells (RBCs) the only thing that can cause shock?

some point, becomes irreversible. Shock is truly "death in progress," so urgent intervention is needed quickly.

Blood loss is not the only factor that can cause shock. Anything that slows down blood circulation will decrease oxygen delivery to the tissues and can cause shock. In trauma, such causes are distributive shock, cardiogenic shock, and of course, hemorrhagic shock.

What Is Shock?

Oxygen in the blood can only be transported when it is bound to hemoglobin (Hb) in RBCs, and one molecule of Hb can only transport four molecules of oxygen.

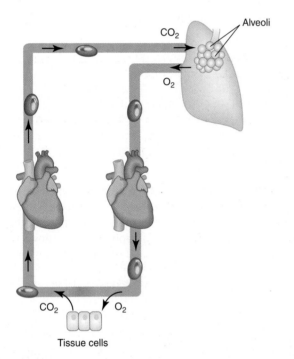

Figure 5-1 The only way for the body to transport more oxygen through the red blood cells is to make the heart beat faster.
© National Association of Emergency Medical Technicians (NAEMT).

The only way for the body to transport more oxygen is to speed up the circulation of RBCs—that is, to make the heart beat faster. If the number of circulating RBCs decreases, so does oxygen transport capacity.

At some point, the remaining blood will not be able to circulate fast enough, and the tissues will not get enough oxygen—that situation is called *shock*.

Every Blood Cell Counts

The Fick principle describes the components necessary for oxygenation of the cells in the body:

- On-loading of oxygen to RBCs in the lung
- Delivery of RBCs to tissue cells
- Off-loading of oxygen from RBCs to tissue cells

- A crucial part of this process is that the patient must have enough RBCs available to deliver adequate amounts of oxygen to tissue cells in order to produce energy.

How Shock Occurs

Cells maintain their normal metabolic functions by producing and using energy in the form of adenosine triphosphate (ATP). The most efficient method of generating energy is through aerobic metabolism. The cells take in oxygen and glucose and metabolize them through a complicated process that produces energy, along with the by-products of water and carbon dioxide.

Anaerobic metabolism, in contrast, occurs without the use of oxygen. It is the backup power system in the body and uses stored body fat as its energy source. Unfortunately, anaerobic metabolism:

- Can run only for a short time
  - Produces 18 times less energy
  - Produces by-products such as lactic acid that are harmful to the body
  - May ultimately become irreversible

If anaerobic metabolism is not corrected quickly, cells start to die, leading to a catastrophic cascade effect. The sensitivity of cells to the lack of oxygen varies from organ system to organ system, and it is greatest in the brain, heart, and lungs.

Shock Kills

Complications of shock include:

- Vascular endothelium damage: resulting in capillary leakage and coagulopathy—onset is in the span of a few minutes
- Renal failure: acute tubular necrosis and anuria—becomes manifest after 6–12 hours
- Bowel ischemia: onset is within several hours, with bacterial translocation and bowel perforation
- Shock lung: occurs within hours, leading to respiratory distress
- Hepatic failure: with coagulopathy, sepsis, multiorgan failure, and death

---

Distracting Causes of Altered Mental Status

The brain is sensitive to both the lack of oxygen and the effects of lactic acidosis, in addition to falling ATP levels.

- Aerobic metabolism produces 36 ATP molecules from 1 glucose and 6 oxygen molecules, along with carbon dioxide and water as waste products.

- Anaerobic metabolism produces 2 ATP molecules per glucose molecule, along with lactic acid as a waste product.

Table 5-1 Organ Tolerance to Ischemia

Organ	Warm Ischemia Time
Heart, brain, lungs	4 to 6 minutes
Kidneys, liver, gastrointestinal tract	45 to 90 minutes
Muscle, bone, skin	4 to 6 hours

Source: American College of Surgeons Committee on Trauma: *Advanced Trauma Life Support for Doctors: Student Course Manual.* 7th ed. Chicago, IL: ACS; 2004.

When the body is in a shock state, it diverts blood flow to save essential organs. That is why less-essential organs that still have a high oxygen need—like the kidneys, liver, lungs, bowel, and vascular endothelium—show damage first, while the heart and brain will be spared to the very end. Anything that slows down the circulation decreases oxygen transport to the tissues and can cause shock. In trauma, such causes are cardiogenic shock, when the heart cannot pump adequately, or distributive shock, where dilation of the vessels diminishes venous return to the heart. However, in the trauma patient, the most frequent cause is hemorrhagic shock, resulting from the loss of circulating blood and decrease in fluid volume.

The Ominous Lactic Acid

In anaerobic metabolism, cells suffering from hypoxia (lack of oxygen) release lactic acid, causing acidosis and respiration increases to "blow off" the acid load. Patients in shock tend to breathe faster, even in the face of perfect lung function.

While not toxic by itself, the accumulation of lactate in the blood is a sure sign that tissues are on an anaerobic diet and that organs are now living on borrowed time.

Transport Early

Emergency medical services (EMS) practitioners have limited means for treating blood loss and shock; thus, rapid transportation to definitive care must be considered early.

FOR MORE INFORMATION

Refer to the "Physiology of Shock" section of Chapter 3: Shock: Pathophysiology of Life and Death.

Identifying Shock

The primary survey of the trauma patient now emphasizes control of life-threatening external bleeding as the first step in the sequence. Assessment and management occur simultaneously, as life threats need to be addressed as soon as they are found (treat as you go):

- **X:** Control any life-threatening external hemorrhage.
- **A:** Make sure the airway is open, especially in unresponsive patients.
- **B:** Optimize ventilation and oxygenation, assisting ventilation if needed. Decompress a tension pneumothorax if needed.
- **C:** If shock is present, organize rapid transport to an appropriate facility. Keep the patient warm, and immobilize major fractures to minimize blood loss. Obtain intravenous (IV) access without delaying transport, and administer tranexamic acid (TXA) and IV fluids if needed while en route.
- **D:** Check for Glasgow Coma Scale (GCS) score and lateralizing signs. Be on the lookout for signs of traumatic brain injury (TBI), because this will influence your treatment.
- **E:** Check for any significant injury you could have missed. Look for contusions and deformations that could indicate internal bleeding.

Control of external hemorrhage should proceed in a stepwise fashion, escalating if initial measures fail to control bleeding.

The Big Picture

Assessing a patient means looking at the big picture—not focusing on a single parameter, such as blood pressure.

How Vital Are Vital Signs?

Exact measurements of vital signs are done just before the secondary survey—they are not necessary to recognize the presence of shock, but they will refine your evaluation and help guide your treatment.

X: External Hemorrhage and Direct Pressure

Why do we check for major bleeding first? Because major bleeding can kill a patient in 3 minutes, and it can be stopped by simple direct pressure. Pressing on the bleeding site long enough allows a clot to form and closes the hole in the vessel. This takes about 3 minutes with a hemostatic dressing and up to 10 minutes with normal gauze (provided the patient is not taking any anticoagulant medications).

The ability of the body to respond to and control bleeding depends on:

- The size of the vessel
  - The pressure within the vessel
  - The presence of clotting factors
  - The ability of the injured vessel to go into spasm and reduce the size of the hole and blood flow at the injury site
  - The pressure of the surrounding tissue on the vessel at the injury site and any additional pressure provided from the outside

Control of external hemorrhage should proceed in a stepwise fashion, escalating if initial measures fail to control bleeding.

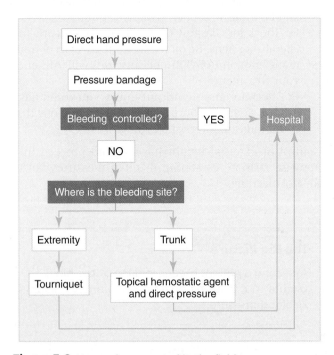

Figure 5-2 Hemorrhage control in the field.
© National Association of Emergency Medical Technicians (NAEMT).

If the dressing becomes soaked with blood, it means that a clot has not formed on the hole in the vessel. Pressure should be maintained because the first clot formed by platelets can only hold a pressure of about 80 mm Hg (the infamous "pop-a-clot" pressure). If the patient's blood pressure is greater than that, the clot will "pop," and bleeding will resume as soon as you let go. Once the bleeding stops, apply a pressure dressing without releasing pressure until the pressure dressing is complete.

PROGRESSIVE CASE STUDY: PART 2

A reassessment of the primary survey finds the following:

- **X:** Bleeding controlled with manual pressure
- **A:** Helmet removed, trauma chin lift to open airway
- **B:** Fast with equal chest rise and clear breath sounds
- **C:** Rapid, thready radial pulse
- **D:** Regaining consciousness, moving all extremities
- **E:** Covered to maintain normothermia

Questions:

- What are the life threats identified?
- Is the patient in shock?
- Why do we check for major bleeding first?
- What is your first move in the face of external hemorrhage?
- How does direct pressure ideally work?
- What if the dressing becomes soaked with blood?
- When would you use a tourniquet in the civilian setting?
- Can pressure be released once the bleeding has stopped?
- How does a tourniquet work?
- Why is a tourniquet applied so tightly?
- Where should the tourniquet be applied and why?
- Would a tourniquet be an option in this patient?
- What are the special considerations?

Tourniquet Use and Occlusive Dressings

Major exsanguination is the quickest way to die. If you are dealing with a hole in the vessel that is too big to be closed by direct pressure, you need to close the vessel by some other means. That is where a tourniquet comes in.

When properly applied, a tourniquet compresses the tissue around the vessel to stop the bleeding. Apply it high and tight above the bleeding site (the goal is to close the vessel, not to compress the bleeding site).

Compressing tissue and muscle requires a lot of pressure, so the tourniquet should be applied tightly enough to block arterial flow and occlude the distal pulse. If one tourniquet does not completely stop the hemorrhage, apply another one just proximal to the first. Once applied, the tourniquet should be left in place until it is no longer needed. The site should not be covered so it can be easily seen and monitored.

Don't Pop That Clot!

Under normal conditions, a platelet clot can hold a pressure of 80 mm Hg, which is enough for most minor wounds. This has two implications for shock treatment.

1. When you stop the bleeding with direct pressure, pressure should be maintained. Otherwise, if your patient's blood pressure is anything more than 80 mm Hg, the clot will "pop" and bleeding will resume.
2. When you face ongoing (internal) bleeding, if you restore normal blood pressure, you will pop any clot that formed at the bleeding site, increasing bleeding. This is why you should not administer a fluid bolus, because this may "overshoot" the target blood pressure range, resulting in recurrent intrathoracic, intra-abdominal, or retroperitoneal bleeding. Titrate your IV fluids!

Three Critical Reminders

- When managing a wound with an impaled object, apply pressure on either side of the object rather than over the object. Impaled objects should not be removed in the field because removal of the object could result in uncontrolled internal hemorrhage.
- If hands are required to perform other lifesaving tasks, you can create a pressure (compression) dressing using gauze pads and an elastic roller bandage or a blood pressure cuff inflated until hemorrhage stops. This dressing is placed directly over the bleeding site.
- Applying direct pressure to exsanguinating hemorrhage takes precedence over insertion of IV lines and fluid resuscitation.

Tourniquet Techniques

- You should apply a tourniquet tight enough to block arterial flow and occlude the distal pulse.
- If one tourniquet does not completely stop the hemorrhage, another one should be applied just proximal to the first.
- Once applied, the tourniquet site should not be covered so it can be easily seen and monitored.
- Once applied, the tourniquet should be left in place until it is no longer needed.

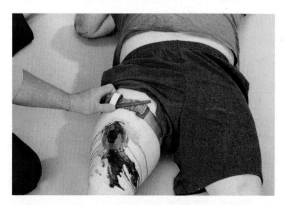

Figure 5-3 Place the tourniquet high and tight.
© Jones & Bartlett Learning. Photographed by Darren Stahlman.

Don't Put the Squeeze On

- A tourniquet cannot be applied to junctional wounds. A special junctional tourniquet is required.
- An occlusive dressing should be considered for a neck wound to prevent air embolism in the event there is a jugular vein injury.

FOR MORE INFORMATION

Refer to the "Management" section of Chapter 3: Shock: Pathophysiology of Life and Death.

Types of Traumatic Shock

Anything that slows down the circulation will decrease oxygen transport to the tissues and can cause shock. In trauma, such causes are shown in Table 5-2.

QUICK TIP

When in doubt, always consider hypovolemic shock as the cause as there is always some degree of hemorrhage in trauma patients.

Table 5-2 Types of Traumatic Shock

	Hypovolemic Shock	Cardiogenic Shock	Distributive Shock
Occurs in/due to	Loss of circulating volume	Impaired cardiac function	Abnormal dilation of the vascular compartment
	■ Blood loss (hemorrhagic shock) ■ Plasma loss (burn patients)	■ Tension pneumothorax ■ Pericardial tamponade ■ Cardiac contusion	High spinal cord injury
Skin temperature/quality	Cool, clammy	Cool, clammy	Warm, dry
Skin color	Pale, cyanotic	Pale, cyanotic	Pink
Blood pressure	Drops	Drops	Drops
Level of consciousness	Altered	Altered	Lucid
Capillary refill time	Slowed	Slowed	Normal

© National Association of Emergency Medical Technicians (NAEMT).

Use Your Tools

Determine the cause of shock through assessment and vital signs:

■ Unequal breath sounds when assessing the patient's breathing may indicate a tension pneumothorax.
■ Blunt chest trauma with electrocardiogram (ECG) changes may indicate a cardiac contusion.
■ High paraplegia or tetraplegia may indicate loss of vascular tone due to the neurologic injury.

Classes of Hemorrhage

Hemorrhagic shock is by far the most frequent cause of shock. The average 150-pound (70-kg) adult human has approximately 5 liters of circulating blood volume. Hemorrhagic shock (hypovolemic shock resulting from blood loss) is categorized into four classes, depending on the severity and amount of blood loss.

Class I Hemorrhage

Class I hemorrhage is compensated shock, as the body can compensate for the lack of oxygen by increasing

Table 5-3 Classification of Hemorrhagic Shock

	Class I	Class II	Class III	Class IV
Blood loss (ml)	< 750	750–1,500	1,500–2,000	> 2,000
Blood loss (% blood volume)	< 15%	15–30%	30–40%	> 40%
Pulse rate	< 100	100–120	120–140	> 140
Blood pressure	Normal	Normal	Decreased	Decreased
Pulse pressure (mm Hg)	Normal or increased	Decreased	Decreased	Decreased
Ventilatory rate	14–20	20–30	30–40	> 35

Table 5-3 Classification of Hemorrhagic Shock (*Continued*)

	Class I	Class II	Class III	Class IV
Central nervous system/mental status	Slightly anxious	Mildly anxious	Anxious, confused	Confused, lethargic
Fluid replacement	Crystalloid	Crystalloid	Crystalloid and blood	Crystalloid and blood

Note: The values and descriptions for the criteria listed for these classes of shock should not be interpreted as absolute determinants of the class of shock, as significant overlap exists.

Source: From American College of Surgeons (ACS) Committee on Trauma. *Advanced Trauma Life Support for Doctors: Student Course Manual.* 8th ed. Chicago, IL: ACS; 2008.

the heart rate and vascular tone (vasoconstriction). The patient is still conscious, the skin is being perfused, urine output is normal, and the ventilatory rate is normal as there is no anaerobic metabolism to create lactic acid in the blood. The release of adrenaline is the cause of the patient being slightly anxious.

Class II Hemorrhage

Class II hemorrhage may result in postural hypotension (i.e., systolic pressure drops when supine). Decreased pulse pressure is due to vasoconstriction and the compensatory mechanism of the body as a result of blood loss.

Class III Hemorrhage

Class III hemorrhage is progressing decompensated shock. If it is not reversed, it will result in multiple organ system failure, and the patient will die. Decreased blood pressure is a late sign. Increasing ventilatory rate is a compensatory mechanism to reverse the effects of lactic acidosis.

Class IV Hemorrhage

Class IV hemorrhage is a stage of severe shock characterized by marked tachycardia (heart rate greater than 120 to 140 beats/min), tachypnea (ventilatory rate greater than 35 breaths/min), profound confusion or lethargy—which means that even the brain is not getting enough oxygen—and greatly decreased systolic blood pressure, typically in the range of 60 mm Hg.

Significant internal hemorrhage can occur with fractures. Fractures of the femur and pelvis are of greatest concern. A single fracture of the femur may be associated

with up to 2 to 4 units (1,000 to 2,000 ml) of blood loss into a thigh. This injury alone could potentially result in the loss of 30% to 40% of an adult's blood volume, resulting in decompensated hypovolemic shock.

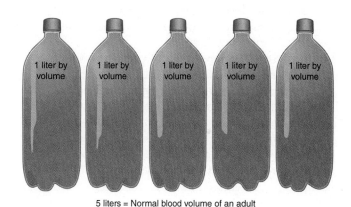

5 liters = Normal blood volume of an adult

Figure 5-4 The approximate amount of blood loss in an adult.
© Jones & Bartlett Learning.

CRITICAL-THINKING QUESTION

Would the patient's pulse oximetry be reliable at this point?

Pulse oximetry relies on pulsatile flow of blood in the capillaries, so diminished blood flow and loss of RBCs render pulse oximetry unreliable. Look at the patient, and do not depend on gadgets that may not be reliable due to decreased blood pressure and decreased peripheral circulation!

Special Populations

Numerous factors can complicate the assessment of the trauma patient, hiding or blunting the usual signs of shock. These factors may mislead the unwary prehospital care provider into thinking a trauma patient is stable when in fact he or she is not. Keep the following in mind:

- **Children:** Children and young adults have a tremendous ability to compensate for blood loss and may appear relatively normal on a quick scan. A closer look may reveal subtle signs of shock, such as mild tachycardia and tachypnea, pale skin with delayed capillary refilling time, and anxiety. Because of their powerful compensatory mechanisms, children found in decompensated shock represent dire emergencies.
- **Geriatric patients:** Geriatric patients often take medications like beta blockers or have pacemakers, so that compensatory tachycardia will be limited or even absent. And a "normal" blood pressure can be lower than the patient's usual blood pressure
- **Pregnant women:** Pregnant women have an increased blood volume (up to 50%), so they can lose a lot of blood before it becomes manifest.
- **Athletes:** Well-trained athletes can have a very low resting heart rate—down to 30–40 beats/min. A rate of 90 beats/min can be a compensatory tachycardia, which can be misinterpreted as a normal value.

FOR MORE INFORMATION

For more information on the anatomy and physiology of shock, refer to the "Assessment" section of Chapter 3: Shock: Pathophysiology of Life and Death.

CRITICAL-THINKING QUESTION

Is it always that easy to tell one shock form from another?

Unfortunately not, as the different shock forms can be present at the same time. For example, a patient with a stab wound to the chest can have cardiogenic shock from a tension pneumothorax and hemorrhagic shock from a leak in the aorta. Be aware, however, that some degree of hemorrhagic shock will almost always be present.

QUICK TIP

Some medications to know when treating shock:	
Beta blockers	Prevent compensatory tachycardia and increase in cardiac output. Interfere with compensatory mechanisms and make evaluation difficult
Antihypertensive drugs	Interfere with compensatory vasoconstriction
Diuretics	Diminish circulating volume so that the patient may be often hypovolemic to begin with
Anticoagulants	Impair function of coagulation factors, so that administration of factors will be necessary
Antiaggregants	Render platelets ineffective, so that platelet transfusion will be needed

FOR MORE INFORMATION

Refer to the "Confounding Factors" section of Chapter 3: Shock: Pathophysiology of Life and Death.

A and B: Airway and Breathing

Once bleeding is controlled, the next priority is to optimize airway and ventilation. Shock is about oxygen transport, so if blood is not correctly oxygenated, every other effort is wasted.

Patients in need of immediate management of their airway include, in order of importance:

- Patients who are not breathing
  - Patients who have obvious airway compromise
  - Patients who have ventilation rates greater than 20 breaths/min
  - Patients who have noisy sounds of ventilation

Advanced techniques for securing the airway and maintaining ventilation may be required in the prehospital setting. Remember to check for pneumothorax; it is the easiest to treat.

QUICK TIP

When anaerobic metabolism kicks in, the brain's sensing system detects the abnormal increase in the amount of carbon dioxide, and it stimulates the respiratory center to increase the rate and depth of ventilation to remove the carbon dioxide. Tachypnea is frequently one of the earliest signs of anaerobic metabolism and shock—even earlier than increased pulse rate. Any pulse oximeter reading below 94% (at sea level) is worrisome and should serve as a stimulus to identify the cause of hypoxia.

C: Circulation

When checking circulation, you need to determine:

- Hemorrhage and the amount of blood loss
  - Perfusion with oxygenated blood
    - Total body
    - Regional

Loss of a radial pulse indicates severe hypovolemia (or vascular damage to the arm), especially when a central pulse is weak, thready, and extremely fast. The exact blood pressure reading is much less important in the primary survey than other, earlier signs of shock.

QUICK TIP

Trauma patients with a weak radial pulse are 15 times more likely to die than patients with a normal pulse.

In addition to the presence of hypoxia and poor perfusion, altered mental status suggests TBI. The combination of hypoxia or decreased blood pressure and TBI has a huge negative impact on patient survival, so hypoxia and hypotension must be corrected or prevented from developing.

Skin that is cool to the touch indicates vasoconstriction, decreased cutaneous perfusion, and decreased energy production and shock. The trauma patient in shock from hypovolemia typically has clammy (moist, diaphoretic) skin. In contrast, the patient with hypotension from a spinal cord injury usually has dry skin.

Once you determine that the victim is in shock, the next priority is timely transport to an adequate surgical facility.

Shock and Skin Color

- Pink skin color generally indicates a well-oxygenated patient without anaerobic metabolism.
- Blue (cyanotic) or mottled skin indicates unoxygenated hemoglobin and a lack of adequate oxygenation to the periphery.
- Pale, mottled, or cyanotic skin has inadequate blood flow resulting from one of the following:
  - Peripheral vasoconstriction (most often associated with hypovolemia)
  - Decreased supply of RBCs (acute anemia)
  - Interruption of blood supply to that portion of the body, such as might be found with a fracture or injury of a blood vessel

---

D: Disability

The brain's ability to function decreases as perfusion and oxygenation drop. Anxiety and belligerent behavior are usually the first signs, followed by a slowing of the thought processes and a decrease of the body's motor and sensory functions.

There are no unique, specific interventions for altered mental status in the shock patient. Assessing a patient's GCS score while still in shock may result in overly grim findings.

Basic Shock Treatment

- Control of external hemorrhage
- Immobilization
- Pelvic binder
- Protect from hypothermia
- Check that external bleeding is stopped

PROGRESSIVE CASE STUDY: PART 3

A reassessment of the primary survey finds:

- **X:** External bleeding still controlled by direct pressure
- **A:** Patent
- **B:** 24 breaths/min, good chest rise, clear equal breath sounds, Spo₂ 97% on oxygen
- **C:** 110 beats/min at carotid and radial; skin cool
- **D:** Conscious, GCS score: 15 (E4, V5, M6), moves all extremities
- **E:** Abrasion and bruising noted to left upper quadrant (LUQ). The patient is complaining of pain 6/10 to his LUQ; however, pain medication is contraindicated at this point due to the patient's blood pressure.

Questions:

- What is the patient's blood pressure, given the vital signs?
- Why is the patient breathing rapidly?
- What are the life threats at this point?
- Why is it important to check the airway and breathing in this patient?
- What signs of shock are present in this patient?
- Is there a possibility of internal bleeding?
- What is "damage control" resuscitation in trauma?
- What happens in the body if we lose blood?
- Can the organs work without oxygen?
- Which organs will become damaged first? When will they fail?
- How does the body react to blood loss?

CRITICAL-THINKING QUESTION

How do you tell if altered level of consciousness (LOC) is due to shock or TBI?

You cannot always tell at first. But if the blood pressure is 55/30 mm Hg and Spo₂ is 70%, altered LOC can be due to hypotension and hypoxemia. If altered LOC persists once hypotension and hypoxemia have been corrected, you must assume TBI is present and set your hemodynamic objectives accordingly.

E: Expose/Environment

Maintaining the patient's body temperature within a normal range is critically important. As the body cools, clotting is impaired. Ideally, the patient compartment of an ambulance should be kept at 85°F (29°C) or more when transporting a severely injured trauma patient.

Shock Management

Steps in the management of shock include:

- Control any external severe hemorrhage.
  - Ensure oxygenation (adequate airway and ventilation).
  - Identify any hemorrhaging. (Control external bleeding and recognize the likelihood of internal hemorrhage.)
  - Transport the patient to definitive care.
  - Administer fluid or blood therapy when appropriate.

FOR MORE INFORMATION

Refer to the "Types of Traumatic Shock" section of Chapter 3: Shock: Pathophysiology of Life and Death.

Advanced Shock Treatment: Vascular Access

Gaining IV access should not delay transport to the hospital for a severely injured patient. It can be done en route. For patients in shock or with potentially serious injuries, one or preferably two large-bore (18-gauge), short (1-inch [25-mm]) IV catheters should be inserted by percutaneous puncture as time permits.

The preferred site for percutaneous access is a vein of the forearm.

QUICK TIP

Alternative sites for IV access are the veins of the antecubital fossa, the hand, and the upper arm (cephalic vein).

Intraosseous (IO) access is most commonly established in sites such as the distal femur, humeral head, or proximal or distal tibia. Studies show best flow rates are through the humeral head and distal femur sites. Fluid administration via the IO route in an awake patient may be painful.

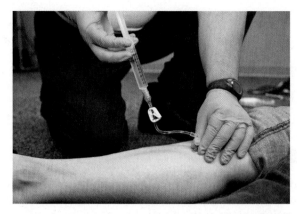

Figure 5-5 IO access may be required to administer fluid.

© National Association of Emergency Medical Technicians (NAEMT).

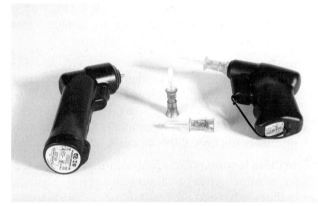

A

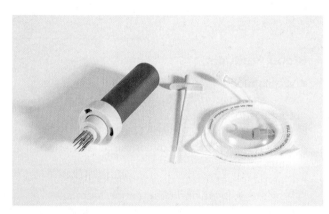

B

Figure 5-6 **A.** IO needles and IO gun for manual insertion (various sizes shown). **B.** IO sternal driver.

© Jones & Bartlett Learning. Photographed by Darren Stahlman.

FOR MORE INFORMATION

Refer to the "Vascular Access" section of Chapter 3: Shock: Pathophysiology of Life and Death.

Fluid Resuscitation

There are two general categories of fluid resuscitation products for the management of trauma patients:

- Blood
  - Packed RBCs (PRBCs)
  - Whole blood
  - Reconstituted whole blood as blood products
  - Plasma
  - Additional blood component therapy
- IV solutions
  - Crystalloid solutions
  - Hypertonic fluid
    - 7% saline
    - 3% saline
  - Colloid solutions
  - Hypotensive or restricted fluid strategies
  - Blood substitutes

Because of its ability to transport oxygen and to clot, blood or various blood products remain the fluid of choice for the resuscitation of a patient in severe hemorrhagic shock.

The rationale for using crystalloids is that since the cardiovascular system is a pump, it needs some volume to work, and crystalloids and colloids can help with that. The downside is dilution of blood components, especially clotting factors, so if you are using crystalloids, only give as much as needed.

The goal of fluid resuscitation is to improve perfusion—restoring a radial pulse and improving mentation.

Know Your Fluids

- Crystalloid isotonic fluids act as effective volume expanders for a short time, but they do not carry oxygen.
  - NaCl 0.9% (normal saline, or NS)
  - Lactated Ringer solution
    - Same amount of sodium as plasma; provides 1:3 volume expansion (2/3 will exit into the extravascular space)
- Colloids are big molecules that will stay in the intravascular compartment; provides 1:1 volume expansion.
  - Hextend
  - Hetastarch
- Blood products provide 1:1 volume expansion, transport oxygen to the tissues, and prevent coagulopathy.
  - Plasma
  - Whole blood

Titrating Trauma Fluid Resuscitation in the Field

- Avoid "popping the clot."
- Superficial wounds do not require immediate IV access or fluid resuscitation.
- If the patient has appropriate mental status and palpable radial pulse, venous access should be limited to a saline lock.
- If the patient has poor mental status or absent radial pulse, IV access and 250-ml bolus should be administered.
  - Continue to repeat bolus if no response.
  - Discontinue fluids to a saline lock if a response is noted.
- Patients with head injuries should have fluids titrated to systolic blood pressure > 90 mm Hg.

Managing Volume in Patients With Signs of Shock and Ongoing Bleeding

- Give just enough fluid to maintain perfusion; that is, until you get a radial pulse or a blood pressure of 80–90 mm Hg systolic.
  - If no signs of shock are present, administer TXA.

QUICK TIP

Remember that a platelet clot can hold up to 80 mm Hg of pressure. If the pressure exceeds this value, all clots already formed inside the body will pop, and bleeding will increase further. A pressure of 80 mm Hg should maintain adequate perfusion to the kidneys with less risk of worsening internal hemorrhage.

- If systolic BP < 80 mm Hg or absent radial pulse, titrate fluid to have a radial pulse or a systolic blood pressure of 80–90 mm Hg (mean arterial pressure [MAP] about 65) and administer TXA when possible.
- In patients with head trauma, titrate fluids to a systolic blood pressure of 100 mm Hg or a MAP or 90 mm Hg.

QUICK TIP

Any IV fluid given to a patient in shock should be warm, not room temperature or cold. The ideal temperature for such fluids is 102°F (39°C).

Blood Products

Blood products offer many advantages. They can restore blood volume, oxygen-carrying capacity, and clotting ability of the blood.

The objectives of blood resuscitation are the restoration of blood volume to restore cellular perfusion but not necessarily restoration of normal blood pressure. The objectives of resuscitation are not the same in every situation.

- In penetrating trauma with hemorrhage, delaying aggressive fluid resuscitation until definitive control may prevent additional bleeding.
- In patients with TBI, a systolic pressure of 100 mm Hg should be achieved to maintain perfusion of the injured brain, even if this means increased bleeding.

While there is widespread agreement that blood transfusion is more efficient, it presents major logistical issues that are beyond the reach of many EMS systems, although technical advances might change this in the near future.

Blood Products

- Whole blood: Provides endothelial cells for oxygen transport as well as platelets and coagulation factors
- RBC concentrates: Provide volume and RBCs for oxygen transport. Do not contain coagulation factors.
- Plasma (never frozen or lyophilized plasma): Provides volume and coagulation factors. Lyophilized plasma is the most practical product to handle to date.

QUICK TIP

Blood and blood products are the gold standard as no other IV fluid can carry oxygen and provide clotting factors.

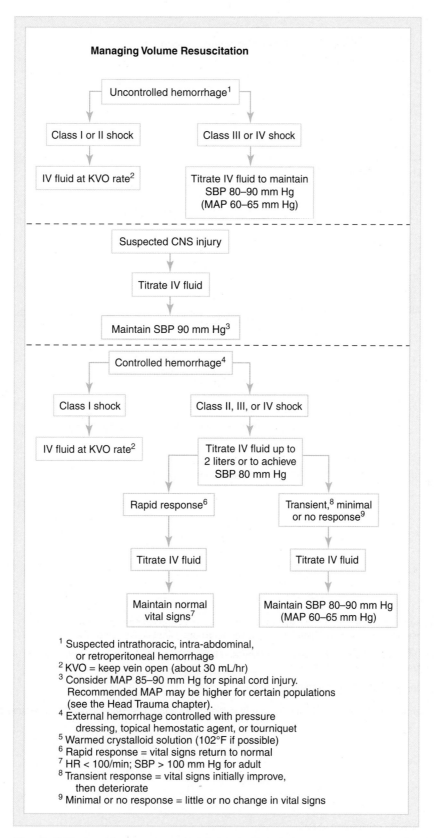

Managing Volume Resuscitation

Uncontrolled hemorrhage[1]

Class I or II shock

Class III or IV shock

IV fluid at KVO rate[2]

Titrate IV fluid to maintain
SBP 80–90 mm Hg
(MAP 60–65 mm Hg)

Suspected CNS injury

Titrate IV fluid

Maintain SBP 90 mm Hg[3]

Controlled hemorrhage[4]

Class I shock

Class II, III, or IV shock

IV fluid at KVO rate[2]

Titrate IV fluid up to
2 liters or to achieve
SBP 80 mm Hg

Rapid response[6]

Transient,[8] minimal
or no response[9]

Titrate IV fluid

Titrate IV fluid

Maintain normal
vital signs[7]

Maintain SBP 80–90 mm Hg
(MAP 60–65 mm Hg)

[1] Suspected intrathoracic, intra-abdominal,
   or retroperitoneal hemorrhage
[2] KVO = keep vein open (about 30 mL/hr)
[3] Consider MAP 85–90 mm Hg for spinal cord injury.
   Recommended MAP may be higher for certain populations
   (see the Head Trauma chapter).
[4] External hemorrhage controlled with pressure
   dressing, topical hemostatic agent, or tourniquet
[5] Warmed crystalloid solution (102°F if possible)
[6] Rapid response = vital signs return to normal
[7] HR < 100/min; SBP > 100 mm Hg for adult
[8] Transient response = vital signs initially improve,
   then deteriorate
[9] Minimal or no response = little or no change in vital signs

Figure 5-7 Algorithm for managing fluid resuscitation.

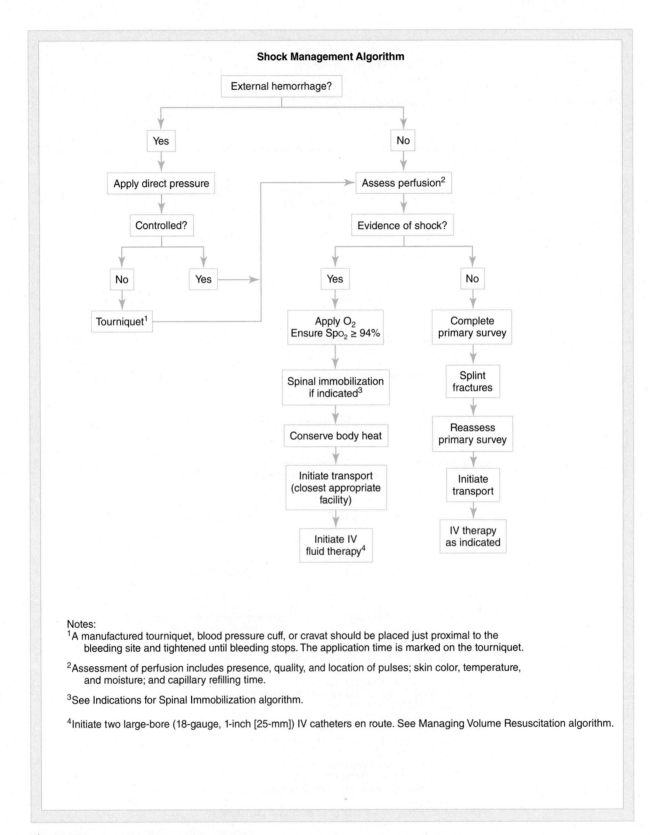

Shock Management Algorithm

Notes:
[1] A manufactured tourniquet, blood pressure cuff, or cravat should be placed just proximal to the bleeding site and tightened until bleeding stops. The application time is marked on the tourniquet.

[2] Assessment of perfusion includes presence, quality, and location of pulses; skin color, temperature, and moisture; and capillary refilling time.

[3] See Indications for Spinal Immobilization algorithm.

[4] Initiate two large-bore (18-gauge, 1-inch [25-mm]) IV catheters en route. See Managing Volume Resuscitation algorithm.

Figure 5-8 Algorithm for managing shock.

Tranexamic Acid

TXA is a clot-stabilizing medication (or antifibrinolytic agent) that has been used for years to control bleeding. It has started to make its way into the prehospital environment. The properties of TXA include:

- It does not promote new clot formation.
- It prevents forming clots from being broken down by the body.

TXA helps reduce blood loss from internal hemorrhage sites that cannot be addressed by tourniquets and hemostatic dressings. It works by binding to plasminogen and preventing it from becoming plasmin, preventing the breakdown of fibrin in a clot. Ongoing studies are needed to determine the appropriate prehospital role for TXA. TXA is supplied in 1-gram (1,000 mg) ampules. You can inject 1 gram of TXA into a 100-ml bag of normal saline or lactated Ringer solution and infuse this volume slowly over 10 minutes.

A second dose, if needed, is typically administered at the hospital, but it may be given if transport times are delayed or long.

WARNING!

Rapid IV push may cause hypotension.

If there is a new-onset drop in blood pressure during the infusion, *slow it down*!

TXA Side Effects

TXA side effects include:

- Nausea, vomiting, diarrhea
- Visual disturbances
- Possible increase in risk of post-injury blood clots
- Hypotension is possible if given too rapidly as an IV bolus

---

CRITICAL-THINKING QUESTIONS

What does rapid transport mean?

It means rapidly assessing and packaging the patient to transport the patient quickly to the appropriate facility (trauma center). The goal is to have an on-scene time of less than 10 minutes.

Should you delay transport to obtain IV access?

No, delaying transport to start an IV is futile. Obtaining IV access can be done during transport; an 18-gauge or larger IV is desirable for blood administration.

What are the components of basic shock treatment? Are they important?

Bleeding control, oxygenation, and maintaining normothermia are all important.

FOR MORE INFORMATION

Refer to the "Volume Resuscitation" section of Chapter 3: Shock: Pathophysiology of Life and Death.

Hypothermia

Coagulopathy, acidosis, and hypothermia are frequently described as the Triad of Death. They are markers of anaerobic metabolism and loss of energy production, and interventions must happen quickly.

Cells work within a finite range of temperature, nominally 98.6°F (37°C). If a patient becomes hypothermic, there is increased oxygen demand for the cells to maintain normal temperature (such as shivering).

Hypothermia is a concern because it affects cellular functions and clotting is diminished. In the field, be sure to maintain normothermia, including keeping the patient covered even when exposing to complete an assessment.

Risk Factors for Hypothermia

- Age: Geriatric and pediatric patients have less effective thermoregulation, thus they are more susceptible to hypothermia.
- Alcohol consumption: Causes vasodilation, increasing heat loss by radiation, and diminishing muscle tone that decreases shivering
- Environment: Immersion in water, cold weather, reduced wind chill, etc.
- Medications: Some medications can affect thermoregulation.
- Mentation: Patients with altered mentation, such as Alzheimer disease, may wander and get lost.
- Physiology: Impairments to thermoregulation, increased heat loss, and problems with heat production

PROGRESSIVE CASE STUDY: SUMMARY

A secondary survey was completed during transport, and the patient was transported to a level I trauma center.

Once in the trauma center, the patient was found to have a ruptured spleen with internal bleeding. He undergoes a surgical splenectomy and makes a good recovery after 5 days in the hospital.

Critical Actions:

The critical actions of the case were:

- Circulation assessment to identify potential life threats
- Determining the best method to manage perfusion in this patient
- Reassessment of perfusion status after initial management was completed

LESSON WRAP-UP

- Stop the bleeding! No IV fluid is better than the patient's blood.
- Use the primary survey to identify life threats.
- Optimize oxygenation.
- Evaluate the need for volume replacement.
- Maintain normothermia.
- You cannot stop internal bleeding in the field—rapid transport is paramount.

PROGRESSIVE CASE STUDY RECAP

Part 1	
Is the patient in shock?	Yes, given the mechanism of injury, altered mental status, and rapid pulse.
What is the definition of shock?	Inadequate cellular perfusion; cells are not receiving oxygen and glucose is needed to create energy.
Why is it so time sensitive?	The lack of oxygen supply to the cells leads to anaerobic metabolism within a few minutes.
What is special about oxygen transport in the blood?	Oxygen binds to hemoglobin on the RBCs.
Is loss of RBCs the only thing that can cause shock?	No, any mechanism that impedes oxygen delivery to the cells can cause shock, such as tension pneumothorax or cardiac tamponade.
Part 2	
What are the life threats identified?	External bleeding, which is controlled, and possible internal bleeding.
Is the patient in shock?	Given the mechanism of injury and the possibility of internal injuries and bleeding, the patient is at risk of shock even though there may not be signs of it currently.
Why do we check for major bleeding first?	Major bleeding can kill a person in 3 minutes, and it can be stopped by simple direct pressure. This is different from hospital ABCDE, because patients with major external bleeding will never arrive in the hospital if the problem is not fixed in the field.

What is your first move in the face of external hemorrhage?	Your first move is direct pressure to the wound, then move to a tourniquet (only if direct pressure does not work).
How does direct pressure ideally work?	By pressing on the bleeding site long enough for a clot to form and close the hole in the vessel. This will take about 3 minutes with a hemostatic dressing and up to 10 minutes with normal gauze, provided the patient is not taking any anticoagulant medications.
What if the dressing becomes soaked with blood?	Bleeding is continuing, and a clot has not formed on the hole in the vessel.
Can pressure be released once the bleeding has stopped?	No! The first clot is formed from platelets that can only hold a blood pressure of about 80 mm Hg (that is the so-called pop-a-clot pressure). If the patient's blood pressure is greater than 80 mm Hg, the clot will pop, and bleeding will resume as soon as you let go.
When would you use a tourniquet in the civilian setting?	When there is severe bleeding from an extremity that cannot be stopped with direct pressure (the hole in the vessel is too big to be controlled by direct pressure).
How does a tourniquet work?	When properly applied, a tourniquet compresses the tissue around the vessel to stop bleeding from the hole in the vessel.
Why is a tourniquet applied so tightly?	Compressing tissue and muscles requires a lot of pressure, which a tourniquet can provide.
Where should the tourniquet be applied and why?	Apply it high and tight above the bleeding site (the goal is to close the vessel, not to compress the bleeding site).
Would a tourniquet be an option in this patient?	No, a tourniquet would not work in this case because the wound is to the anterior neck.
What are the special considerations?	A tourniquet cannot be applied to junctional wounds; a special junctional tourniquet is required.
	An occlusive dressing should be considered for the neck wound to prevent air embolism in the event there is a jugular vein injury.
Part 3	
What is the patient's blood pressure, given the vital signs?	At least 80–90 mm Hg because there is a radial pulse.
Why is the patient breathing rapidly?	It could be a result of the stress of the situation, and it could also be due to shock from blood loss (rapid breathing compensating for lactic acid production).
What are the life threats at this point?	The abrasion and hematoma to the LUQ may indicate internal bleeding.
Why is it important to check the airway and breathing in this patient?	If there is no airway and breathing, then oxygen is not being carried by the blood. Given the mechanism of injury, it is important to rule out other injuries, such as tension pneumothorax (which is easily treated).

(continued)

PROGRESSIVE CASE STUDY RECAP (*CONTINUED*)

What signs of shock are present in this patient?	Rapid breathing, rapid heart rate, cool skin (also low blood pressure, if assessed)
Is there a possibility of internal bleeding?	There is a high probability given the mechanism of injury, the abrasion and bruising to the LUQ, and the signs of shock.
What is "damage control" resuscitation in trauma?	Body rewarming, restrictive fluid administration, permissive hypotension, blood product administration, and execution of transfusion products
What happens in the body if we lose blood?	The capacity of the cardiovascular system to transport oxygen is reduced.
Can the organs work without oxygen?	Yes; however, without oxygen, the organs switch to anaerobic metabolism, which produces 18 times less energy.
Which organs will become damaged first? When will they fail?	Unlike in cardiac arrest, the body will be able to save circulation for the most essential organs; that is, the brain and the heart, to the expense of tissues with low oxygen requirements like bone or fat. As shock worsens, organs with medium oxygen requirements will begin to be damaged (kidney, lung, liver, vascular endothelium). Even if it is not immediately obvious, it is a time bomb that will detonate in the intensive care unit (ICU) some hours later.
How does the body react to blood loss?	Since there is less oxygen carrying capacity, the body has to make blood run faster; that is, the heart will beat faster. Lactic acid forms from anaerobic metabolism and causes acidosis, which makes the patient breathe faster to compensate for the acidic state.

STUDY QUESTIONS

1. Your patient is a 40-year-old male who has been stabbed multiple times in the left chest. He ran away from his attacker before he collapsed on the sidewalk. He is pale and confused and complains of difficulty breathing. A wound above the left clavicle is bleeding profusely. Your first move is to:
   A. give oxygen and insert an IV.
   B. decompress the left chest.
   C. begin direct compression of the bleeding site.
   D. use a junctional tourniquet.

2. Your partner is compressing the bleeding site. The bleeding seems to be controlled, yet the patient becomes combative. He complains that he can't breathe and that he is about to die. Your next move is to:
   A. start assisted ventilation.
   B. give high-flow oxygen.
   C. decompress the left chest.
   D. give a 250-ml fluid bolus.

3. You have decompressed the chest, and the patient's respiration improves markedly, but he remains confused. He has an absent radial pulse, and his carotid pulse is fast and thready. Your partner asks if he can let the compression go to put in an IV. How should you respond?
   A. "Oh yes, that's a great idea!"
   B. "Yes, but we have to immobilize him first."
   C. "Take a blood pressure first to see if he needs an IV."
   D. "No, keep the pressure and let's get out of here!"

4. While en route to the hospital, you manage to put an 18-gauge IV in the right arm. Your patient is still confused, and you still have no radial pulse. Your next move is to:
   A. give 1-liter fluid bolus.
   B. give one 250-ml fluid bolus then stop.
   C. give fluid until you get a radial pulse.
   D. administer TXA.

5. After 400 ml of lactated Ringer solution, you get a radial pulse and his level of consciousness improves. The monitor shows: heart rate 110 beats/min, blood pressure 85/60 mm Hg, Spo$_2$ 95%, ventilation rate 25 breaths/min. What should you do?
    A. Give an additional 500 ml of lactated Ringer solution.
    B. Stop fluids and give 1 g of TXA.
    C. Give TXA and 500 ml of normal saline.
    D. Give 2 mg of morphine for analgesia.

6. You now perform a secondary survey and SAMPLE. You notice two additional stab wounds medial to the left nipple and a sternotomy scar. Your patient tells you he is on clopidogrel PO since he had a coronary artery bypass graft 2 years ago. Is this information useful?

    A. No, he should stop talking and breathe.
    B. Yes, he should see a cardiologist once in the local hospital.
    C. Yes, he will need platelets and a heart surgeon ASAP.
    D. Yes, you should raise his blood pressure up to 130 mm Hg systolic.

7. Oh, by the way, did you immobilize your patient?
    A. Yes, as I always do.
    B. Yes, because a stab to the trunk could have injured his spinal cord.
    C. Yes, because he might have TBI.
    D. No, it's a waste of time in a patient with stab wounds.

ANSWER KEY

Question 1: C
Stopping life-threatening external bleeding with direct pressure is the priority and can be done quickly. A junctional tourniquet is not the first maneuver because it takes much more time.

Question 2: C
After X come A and B. You can quickly auscultate the lungs (pneumothorax is almost certain with multiple stabs in the chest) and decompress the chest. Decompressing a tension pneumothorax is the quickest way to treat shock.

Question 3: D
This patient is likely in decompensated shock with internal bleeding, so rapid transport is the next priority. You should maintain pressure on the wound, because having massive external bleeding start up again is the last thing you want in this situation.

Question 4: C
Now is the time to titrate IV fluids to restore tissue perfusion. Giving 1 liter blindly could overshoot your target pressure and reinforce internal bleeding. TXA is not a priority, although it can run parallel to fluids.

Question 5: B
The patient does not need more fluids right now. Giving morphine in a shocked patient is a risky move and could lead to dangerous hypotension.

Question 6: C
The stab wound is in the infamous "cardiac box" which puts him at risk of a cardiac injury. Because he is on clopidogrel, his platelets are out of order for at least 5 days, so he will require urgent platelet transfusion.

Question 7: D
In penetrating trauma, you only immobilize if there are signs of spinal lesion, which is not the case here. (He ran away from his attacker, remember?) Spinal immobilization is not indicated, and in this case would be a disastrous waste of time.

REFERENCES AND FURTHER READING

National Association of Emergency Medical Technicians. *PHTLS: Prehospital Trauma Life Support*. 9th ed. Burlington, MA: Public Safety Group; 2019.

SKILL STATIONS

Tourniquet Application

1. Remove the tourniquet from the carrying pouch.
2. Slide the patient's extremity through the loop of the self-adhering band, or wrap the self-adhering band around the extremity and reattach it to the friction adapter buckle.
3. Position the tourniquet as high as possible on the limb.
4. Secure the tourniquet. If applying to a leg wound, the self-adhering band must be routed through both sides of the friction adapter buckle and fastened back on itself. This will prevent it from loosening when twisting the windlass clip or tri-ring (per the device's guidelines and only applicable to some tourniquets).
5. Twist the windlass rod until the bleeding stops. Ensure that the distal pulse is no longer palpable.
6. Lock the rod in place with the windlass clip or tri-ring. *Note: For added security (and always before moving the patient), secure the windlass rod with the windlass strap. For smaller extremities, continue to wind the self-adhering band across the windlass clip and secure it under the windlass strap.*
7. Grasp the windlass strap, pull it tight, and adhere it to the Velcro on the windlass clip (per the device's guidelines).
8. Document time of tourniquet application and document absence of distal pulses.

Junctional Tourniquet Application

1. Determine that the injury is not amenable to treatment with a standard limb tourniquet
2. Cut away the patient's clothing.
3. The remainder of the steps will be per manufacturer's direction, depending on device used. Slide the belt underneath the patient, positioning the target compression device (TCD) over the area to be compressed (over the femoral pulse just below the inguinal ligament). Apply sterile gauze or hemostatic dressing directly over the wound. When treating a unilateral injury and using only one TCD, the belt may be applied from either side, depending on the location of the injury. For bilateral application, use a second TCD.
4. Hold the TCD in place and connect the belt by snapping the buckle together.
5. Pull the brown handles away from each other until the buckle secures. An audible click is heard. Fasten the excess belt in place by pressing it down on the Velcro strap. A second click may be heard once the belt is secure.
6. Use the hand pump to inflate the TCD until hemorrhage stops.
7. Monitor the patient during transport for hemorrhage control, adjusting the device if necessary.*

or

1. Determine that the injury is not amenable to treatment with a standard limb tourniquet.
2. Verbalize cutting away the patient's clothing.
3. Place pressure pads just below the inguinal ligament.
4. Determine if a bilateral or unilateral application is required.
5. Unroll the device in preparation for application.
6. Slide the belt with "This Side Toward Casualty" facing up under the body at the lower back.
7. Locate the superior iliac crest and pubic bone connected by the inguinal ligament.

*SAM junctional tourniquet instructions from: https://www.sammedical.com/assets/uploads/sjt-instructional-poster_2017-04-10.pdf

Wound Packing

1. Expose the injury by opening or cutting away the patient's clothing.
2. If possible, remove excess blood from the wound while preserving any clots that may have formed.
3. Locate the source of the most active bleeding.
4. Remove the hemostatic agent or plain gauze from its sterile package, and pack it tightly into the wound directly over the site of the most active bleeding.
5. More than one gauze roll may be required to control the hemorrhage.
6. Apply direct pressure over the wound, and pack with enough force to stop the bleeding.
7. Hold direct pressure for a minimum of 3 minutes (if using a hemostatic agent and per the manufacturer's instructions) or 10 minutes if using plain gauze.
8. After the required amount of time for application of direct pressure has elapsed, reassess the patient for bleeding control.
9. The wound may be repacked as necessary to stop any continued bleeding. Old packing should not be removed.
10. Leave the wound packing in place and secure it in place with a compression dressing.

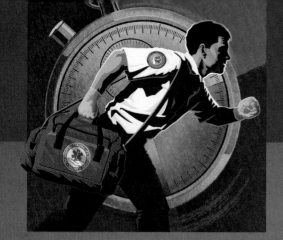

LESSON 6

Secondary Survey

LESSON OBJECTIVES

· Explain the purpose and sequencing of performing a secondary survey.
· Choose the most appropriate secondary survey tool(s) to obtain pertinent physical findings.
· Identify transport options for a trauma patient based on assessment findings.

PROGRESSIVE CASE STUDY: PART 1

It's a Saturday morning in early November. The weather is clear, with an outside temperature of 42°F (5.5°C). You're dispatched to a residential area for a person who has fallen from the roof of a two-story building.

Upon arrival at the scene, you are met by an adult family member who leads you around the house to the backyard. The family member states the patient was cleaning leaves from the rain gutters when he lost his balance and fell approximately 12 ft (3.6 m) from the roof, landing on his back. The patient initially lost consciousness for a "brief period" but was conscious by the time the family member called 9-1-1.

A level II hospital is 10 minutes away by ground. A level I trauma center is 2 hours away by ground and 30 minutes by air; fixed wing is 30 minutes from the scene.

Your scene size-up reveals a ladder laying on the grass. The patient is lying beside the ladder.

Your primary survey reveals the following:

X—No visible signs of hemorrhage
A—Patent, you see no airway obstruction; your partner is holding manual cervical spine stabilization
B—Shallow with diminished lung sounds; 18 breaths/min, unable to take a deep breath due to upper back pain; SpO_2 94%
C—Skin is pink, cool, and dry; pulse 112 beats/min, $ETCO_2$ 40 mm Hg
D—Patient is conscious, confused, Glasgow Coma Scale (GCS) 14 (E4, V4, M6), pupils 3 mm and equal bilaterally
E—Outside temp is cool 42°F (5.5°C). Patient's temperature is 98.4°F (36.8°C).

Questions:

■ For this patient, is the secondary survey performed in the field or during transport?
■ What are the main objectives of the secondary survey?
■ What is the importance of vital signs during the secondary survey?
■ What is the importance of the SAMPLE history during the secondary survey?
■ How would you use "see, hear, feel" to complete the secondary survey?
■ What type of clues can be "heard" during the secondary survey?
■ What could be "heard" that would indicate an injury to the neck?
■ Could a patient's lung sounds lead you to hidden injuries?
■ When "feeling" for injuries on the head, what are your hands telling you?
■ Can you assess ("feel") the patient's neck during the secondary survey?
■ How important is it to "feel" the patient's chest expand during the secondary survey?

Introduction

Assessment is the foundation on which all management and transport decisions are based. You need to establish an overall impression of a patient's status and determine baseline values for the patient's respiratory, circulatory, and neurologic systems. If time and the patient's condition allow, a secondary survey is conducted for non-threatening injuries. Often this secondary survey occurs during patient transport.

It's All in the Timing

Critical patients should not remain in the field for care other than to manage immediate life threats, unless they're trapped, or other complications exist that prevent early transport.

Secondary Survey

Because a well-performed primary survey will identify all immediately life-threatening conditions, the secondary survey, by definition, deals with less serious problems. It's a more detailed head-to-toe evaluation of a patient performed only after the primary survey is completed, all identified life-threatening injuries have been managed, and resuscitation has been initiated. The goal of the secondary survey is to identify injuries or problems that weren't identified during the primary survey.

QUICK TIP

A critical trauma patient is transported as soon as possible after the conclusion of the primary survey and not held in the field for either IV initiation or a secondary survey.

The secondary survey uses a "look, listen, and feel" approach to evaluate the patient. You identify injuries and correlate physical findings region by region, beginning at the head and proceeding through the neck, chest, and abdomen to the extremities, concluding with a detailed neurologic examination.

- See, don't just look.
- Hear, don't just listen.
- Feel, don't just touch.

While examining the patient, use all the available information to formulate a patient care plan.

- See
  - Examine all of the skin of each region.
  - Be attentive for external hemorrhage or signs of internal hemorrhage, such as distension of

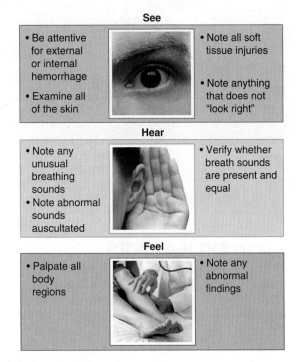

See
- Be attentive for external or internal hemorrhage
- Examine all of the skin
- Note all soft tissue injuries
- Note anything that does not "look right"

Hear
- Note any unusual breathing sounds
- Note abnormal sounds auscultated
- Verify whether breath sounds are present and equal

Feel
- Palpate all body regions
- Note any abnormal findings

Figure 6-1 See, Hear, Feel.
Photos: Eye photo © iStockphoto/Thinkstock; ear photo: © iStockphoto/Thinkstock; hands photo: © Image Point Fr/ShutterStock.
Art: © National Association of Emergency Medical Technicians.

the abdomen, swollen and tense extremity, or an expanding hematoma.
  - Identify soft-tissue injuries, including abrasions, burns, contusions, hematomas, lacerations, and puncture wounds.
  - Note any masses or swelling, or deformation of bones (deformities).
  - Note abnormal indentations on the skin and the skin's color.
  - Note anything that doesn't "look right."
- Hear
  - Note any unusual sounds when the patient inhales or exhales. Normal breathing is quiet.
  - Note any abnormal sounds when auscultating the chest.
  - Check whether the breath sounds are equal in both lung fields.
  - Auscultate over the carotid arteries and note any unusual sounds (bruits) over the vessels that would indicate vascular damage (often not realistic on a trauma scene).
- Feel
  - Firmly palpate all parts of the region, including bones. Note whether:
    - Anything moves that shouldn't
    - There's any crepitus or subcutaneous emphysema
    - The patient complains of tenderness
    - All pulses are present (and where they are felt)
    - Pulsations are felt that should not be present

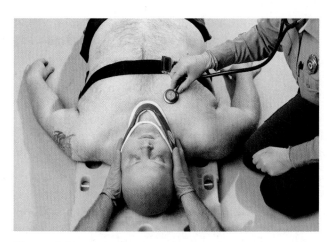

Figure 6-2 Check whether the breath sounds are equal in both lung fields.
© Jones & Bartlett Learning. Photographed by Darren Stahlman.

- Carefully move each joint in the region. Note any resulting crepitus, pain, or limitation of range of motion, or unusual movement, such as laxity.

Remember that a good detailed secondary survey will increase the patient's chance of survival by identifying any issues and reporting them during your transfer of care. Any injury can be missed, or its significance may not have presented, during your rapid primary survey.

> **QUICK TIP**
>
> Be detailed and thorough during your secondary survey, not letting distracting injuries become your pitfall.

> **QUICK TIP**
>
> Be sure to continually assess the patient's heart rate, as tachycardia may be a response to anxiety, pain, temperature, or fear, but also a trending increase in heart rate is a good indicator for ongoing blood loss.

Vital Signs

The first step of the secondary survey is measuring the vital signs. You'll continuously reevaluate the rate and quality of the pulse, rate and depth of ventilation, and the other components of the primary survey and compare them to previous findings because big changes can occur rapidly.

A set of complete vital signs includes:

- Blood pressure
- Pulse rate and quality

- Ventilatory rate and depth
- Oxygen saturation (pulse oximetry)
- Skin color and temperature
- Body temperature

> **QUICK TIP**
>
> Depending on the situation, a second prehospital care provider may obtain vital signs while the first provider completes the primary survey, to avoid further delay.

For the critical trauma patient, you should evaluate and record a complete set of vital signs every 3 to 5 minutes, if possible, and at the time of any change in condition or a medical problem. Even if an automated, noninvasive blood pressure device is available, always take the initial blood pressure manually.

> **QUICK TIP**
>
> Automatic blood pressure devices may be inaccurate when the patient is significantly hypotensive; in these patients, all blood pressure measurements should be obtained manually, or at least confirm correlation of automated reading with manual reading.

Pain Management

Pain should be treated like any other vital sign. Treat any pain associated with a traumatic injury, since pain increases the stress response in the body, which directly affects the patient's other vital signs.

Traditionally, pain management has had a limited role in the management of trauma patients, mostly because of the concern that the side effects of narcotics would aggravate preexisting hypoxia and hypotension, and ketamine can aggravate agitation. This has resulted in pain relief being denied to some patients with appropriate indications (such as an isolated limb injury or spinal fracture). You can consider pain management in such patients, particularly in cases of prolonged transport, as long as the signs of ventilatory impairment or shock aren't present. Providers should follow local pain management protocols.

Monitor pulse oximetry and serial vital signs vigilantly if any narcotics are administered to a trauma patient.

SAMPLE History

Obtain a quick history on the patient and document it on the patient care report to be passed on to the medical personnel at the receiving facility. The mnemonic SAMPLE serves as a reminder of the key components:

- **S**ymptoms: What does the patient complain of? Pain? Trouble breathing? Numbness? Tingling?
- **A**llergies: Does the patient have any known allergies, particularly to medications? Pay careful attention to medically relevant allergies, such as latex, penicillin, and radiology contrast.

- **M**edications: What prescription or nonprescription medications (including vitamins, supplements, and other over-the-counter medications) does the patient regularly take? Any anticoagulants or anti-aggregants, insulin, or beta blockers? What recreational substance does he or she use regularly and, in particular, today?
- **P**ast medical and surgical history: Does the patient have any significant medical problems requiring ongoing medical care? Has the patient undergone any prior surgeries?
- **L**ast meal/Last menstrual period: How long has it been since the patient last ate? Many trauma patients will require surgery, and recent food intake increases the

---

SCENARIO: PART 2

The SAMPLE history reveals the following:

S—Upper and lower back pain
A—Sulfa medications
M—Lisinopril, HCTZ, simvastatin
P—Hypertension, hyperlipidemia
L—Breakfast: coffee and toast
E—Cleaning the rain gutters, standing on the roof
After "searching" for injuries using the "see, hear, feel" approach, the secondary survey shows that the patient has upper and lower back pain. During palpation of the pelvis, the pelvis feels unstable. The patient's neurologic exam is within normal limits.

You take a set of vital signs:

- BP: 106/40 mm Hg
- Heart rate and quality: 112 beats/min, regular and thready at the radial pulse
- Ventilation rate: 18 breaths/min, shallow with diminished lung sounds. Patient states he cannot take a deep breath due to the pain in his upper back.
- Spo$_2$: 94% on room air
- ETCO$_2$: 40 mm Hg
- Glucose: 96 mg/dl (5.3 mmol/l)
- Skin condition and temperature: Pink, warm, and dry
- Temperature: 97°F (36°C)
- Pain: 8/10 to back and pelvis—10/10 on movement and palpation

Questions:
- What injuries may be hidden in the abdomen? More importantly, what injuries may NOT be hidden in the abdomen?
- Why should palpation of the pelvis be done with caution?
- What injuries might we find while "feeling" the extremities of this patient?
- When and how frequently should you calculate the patient's GCS?
- What can you tell from "looking into someone's eyes"?
- How often should you assess the patient's motor and sensory function?

risk of aspiration during induction of anesthesia. For female patients of childbearing age, when was their last menstrual period? Is there a possibility of pregnancy?

- **E**vents: What events preceded the injury? Immersion in water (drowning or hypothermia) and exposure to hazardous materials should be included.

Slow It Down to Speed It Up

Remember that when trying to obtain your SAMPLE history with geriatric patients, they may already be faced with communication issues (hearing and speech) as a result of the aging process. While you may be in a hurry for answers due to the traumatic event, you may need to slow down and speak up, allowing the older patient time to process the question and respond.

FOR MORE INFORMATION

Refer to the "Secondary Survey" section of Chapter 6: Patient Assessment and Management.

Examining Anatomic Regions

Head

Visually examine the head and face for contusions, abrasions, lacerations, bone asymmetry, hemorrhage, bony

defects of the face and supportive skull, and abnormalities of the eye, eyelid, external ear, mouth, and mandible.

Steps during a head examination include:

- Search thoroughly through the patient's hair for any soft-tissue injuries.
- Check pupil size for reactivity to light, equality, roundness, and irregular shape.
- Carefully palpate the bones of the face and skull to identify focal tenderness, crepitus, deviation, depression, or abnormal mobility. (This is extremely important in the nonradiographic evaluation for head injury.)
- Be careful when attempting to open and examine the eyes of an unconscious trauma patient who has evidence of facial injury. Even small amounts of pressure may further damage an eye that has a blunt or penetrating injury.
- Check for bruising around the eyes (racoon eye) and behind the ears (Battle's sign); however, these are late findings that appear many hours after the injury.
- Check for blood or fluid draining from the ears and nose.

QUICK TIP

Fractures of the bones of the midface are often associated with a fracture of the portion of the skull base called the cribriform plate. If the patient has midface trauma (e.g., injury between the upper lip and orbits), a gastric tube, if used, should be inserted through the mouth rather than through the nose, due to the risk of intracranial placement.

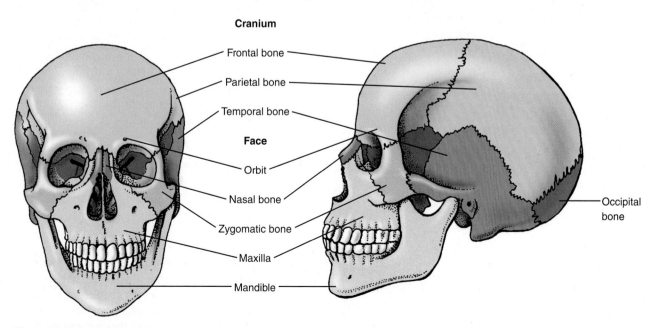

Figure 6-3 Normal anatomic structure of the face and skull.
© National Association of Emergency Medical Technicians.

Neck

Visual examination of the neck for contusions, abrasions, lacerations, hematomas, and deformities will alert you to the possibility of underlying injuries. Palpation may reveal subcutaneous emphysema from a laryngeal, tracheal, or pulmonary origin. Crepitus of the larynx, hoarseness, and subcutaneous emphysema constitute a triad classically indicative of laryngeal fracture. Lack of tenderness of the cervical spine may help rule out cervical spine fractures (when combined with strict criteria), whereas tenderness may indicate the presence of a fracture, dislocation, or ligamentous injury. You need to perform such palpation carefully, making sure that the cervical spine remains in a neutral, in-line position.

Just Because You Can't Find It, Doesn't Mean It Isn't a Problem

Absence of a neurologic deficit does not exclude the possibility of an unstable cervical spine injury. Reevaluation may reveal expansion of a previously identified hematoma or shifting of the trachea.

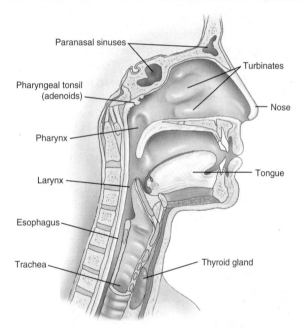

Figure 6-4 Normal anatomy of the neck.
© National Association of Emergency Medical Technicians.

Chest

Because the thorax is strong, resilient, and elastic, it can absorb a significant amount of trauma. You need to do a close visual examination of the chest for deformities, areas of paradoxical movement, contusions, and abrasions to identify underlying injuries. Other signs you need to be aware of include:

* Splinting and guarding
* Unequal bilateral chest excursion

* Intercostal, suprasternal, or supraclavicular bulging or retraction

A contusion over the sternum may be the only indication of an underlying cardiac injury.

Auscultation with a stethoscope is an essential part of the chest examination. A patient will most often be in a supine position so that only the anterior and lateral chest is available for auscultation. It's important to recognize normal and decreased breath sounds with a patient in this position.

* Diminished or absent breath sounds indicate a possible pneumothorax, tension pneumothorax, or hemothorax.
* Crackles heard posteriorly (when the patient is logrolled) or laterally may indicate pulmonary contusion.
* Cardiac tamponade is characterized by distant heart sounds; however, these may be difficult to ascertain given the commotion at the scene or road noise during transport.

A small area of rib fractures may indicate a severe underlying pulmonary contusion. Any type of compression injury to the chest can result in a pneumothorax. The thorax is palpated for the presence of subcutaneous emphysema (air in the soft tissue).

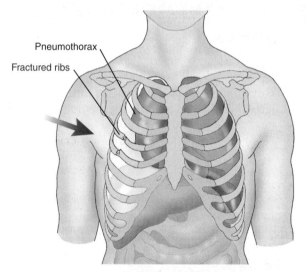

Figure 6-5 Compression injury to the chest can result in rib fracture and subsequent pneumothorax.
© National Association of Emergency Medical Technicians.

QUICK TIP

The chest walls of pediatric patients are thinner and less muscular than that of an adult, so it may be difficult to determine breath sounds based on left versus right since the sounds from one are often heard in the other side, as well. Try listening to the breath sounds just below the armpit on the side; that will help give some distance between the lungs.

Abdomen

The abdominal examination begins with visual evaluation. Abrasions and discoloration indicate the possibility of underlying injury; in particular, periumbilical and flank ecchymosis is associated with retroperitoneal bleeding (however, these are late findings that appear hours after the injury occurred).

> **Interpreting Seat Belt Sign**
>
> In the case of a motor vehicle collision, you should examine the abdomen carefully for a telltale transverse contusion, which initially appears as a red mark across the abdomen and suggests that a seat belt may have caused underlying injury. A significant portion of patients with this sign will have underlying injury, most frequently small bowel injury. Lumbar spine fractures may also be associated with the "seat belt sign."

You'll also need to palpate each quadrant to evaluate for tenderness, abdominal muscle guarding, and masses. When palpating, note whether the abdomen is soft or whether rigidity or guarding is present. There's no need to continue palpating after discovering abdominal tenderness or pain. Additional information won't alter prehospital management, and the only outcomes of a continued abdominal examination are further discomfort to the patient and delayed transport to the receiving facility. The peritoneal cavity can hide a large volume of blood, often with minimal or no abdominal distension.

> **Gut Reactions**
>
> Altered mental status resulting from a traumatic brain injury or intoxication with alcohol or other drugs often obscures evaluation of the abdomen.

Pelvis

First, visually examine the pelvis for abrasions, contusions, hematomas, lacerations, open fractures, and signs of distension. Pelvic fractures can produce massive internal hemorrhage, resulting in rapid deterioration of a patient's hemodynamic status.

Palpation of the pelvis provides minimal information that will affect the management of the patient. Because palpation of the unstable pelvis can move fractured segments and disrupt any blood clot that's formed, this step should be performed only once and not repeated.

Palpation is accomplished by gently applying front-to-back pressure with the heels of the hands on the symphysis pubis and then medial pressure to the iliac crests bilaterally, evaluating for pain and abnormal movement. Stop if you find any evidence of instability and place a pelvic binder or otherwise immobilize the pelvis.

> **Be Hip to Hip Fractures**
>
> When treating older patients with a possible pelvic or femoral neck fracture, this event can lead to a rapid decline in their health and quality of life. Do not treat them as just another limited injury, they will require aggressive medical care and emotional support.

Genitals

In general, genitals are not examined in detail in the prehospital setting. However, you should note any bleeding from the external genitalia, obvious blood at the urethral meatus, or presence of priapism in males. Additionally, clear fluid noted in the pants of a pregnant patient may represent amniotic fluid from rupture of the amniotic membranes, or urinary incontinence if present in any patient.

Back

Examine the back for evidence of injury. This is easier when logrolling the patient for placement onto or removal from the long backboard. You should auscultate breath sounds over the posterior thorax, and observe the back for contusions, abrasions, and deformities. Palpate the spine for tenderness and deformity.

Extremities

The examination of the extremities begins at the clavicle in the upper extremity and the pelvis in the lower extremity and then proceeds toward the most distal portion of each extremity. Evaluate each individual bone and joint by visual inspection for deformity, hematoma, or ecchymosis and by palpation to determine the presence of crepitus, pain, tenderness, or unusual movements. Any suspected fracture should be immobilized. Check circulation and motor and sensory nerve function at the distal end of each extremity.

> QUICK TIP
>
> If an extremity is immobilized, pulses, movement, and sensation should be checked both before and after splinting.

Neurologic Examination

As with the other regional examinations, the neurologic examination in the secondary survey is conducted in much greater detail than in the primary survey and includes:

- Calculation of the Glasgow Coma Scale (GCS)
- Evaluation of motor and sensory function
- Observation of pupillary response

A gross examination of sensory capability and motor response helps determine the presence or absence of weakness or loss of sensation in the extremities, suggesting brain or spinal cord injury, and will identify areas that require further examination.

When examining a patient's pupils, evaluate the equality of response in addition to equality of size.

Eye Opening	Points
Spontaneous eye opening	4
Eye opening on command	3
Eye opening to pressure	2
No eye opening	1
Best Verbal Response	
Answers appropriately (oriented)	5
Gives confused answers	4
Inappropriate words	3
Makes unintelligible noises	2
Makes no verbal response	1
Best Motor Response	
Follows command	6
Localizes	5
Normal flexion response	4
Abnormal flexion response	3
Extension response	2
Gives no motor response	1
Total	

Figure 6-6 GCS.

© Jones & Bartlett Learning.

Windows to the Brain

A small but significant portion of the population has pupils of differing sizes (anisocoria) as a normal condition. Even in these patients, however, the pupils should react to light in a similar manner.

Pupils that react at differing speeds to the introduction of light are considered to be unequal. Unequal pupils in an unconscious trauma patient may indicate increased intracranial pressure or pressure on the third cranial nerve, caused by either cerebral edema or a rapidly expanding intracranial hematoma. Direct eye injury can also cause unequal pupils.

FOR MORE INFORMATION

Refer to the "Assessing Anatomic Regions" section of Chapter 6: Patient Assessment and Management.

Definitive Care in the Field

Definitive care is an intervention that completely corrects a particular condition.

Definitive care for many of the injuries sustained by the critical trauma patient can be provided only in the hospital setting. Anything that delays the administration of that definitive care lessens the patient's chance of survival. Further, while one injury or condition may be definitively treated in the field, most major trauma patients will have multiple injuries that must be treated in the hospital.

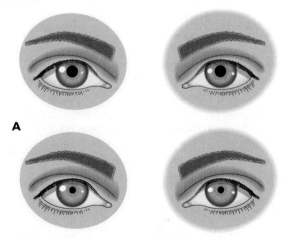

A

C

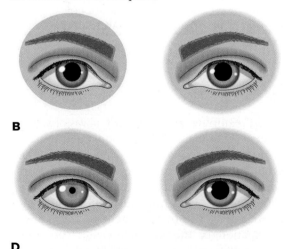

B

D

Figure 6-7 A. Normal pupils. **B.** Pupil dilation. **C.** Pupil constriction. **D.** Unequal pupils.

© Jones & Bartlett Learning.

FOR MORE INFORMATION

Refer to the "Definitive Care in the Field" section of Chapter 6: Patient Assessment and Management.

Transport

Because trauma patients often have spinal injuries, be prepared to stabilize the patient's spine. If there's time, you can stabilize extremity fractures and bandage major wounds.

For some critically injured trauma patients, initiating transport is the single most important aspect of definitive care in the field. A patient whose condition isn't critical can get attention for individual injuries before transport, but even this patient should be transported as soon as possible before a hidden condition becomes critical.

Field Triage

The "where" a patient is transported is also extremely important, and is based on the patient's injuries (or suspected injuries). Studies show better patient outcomes for trauma patients treated at specifically staffed trauma centers.

Location, Location, Location

A study funded by the Centers for Disease Control and Prevention (CDC), published in 2006, demonstrated that patients were 25% more likely to survive their injuries if they received care at a level I trauma center than if they were cared for in a nontrauma center.

CDC Guidelines for Field Triage of Injured Patients

At first glance, the CDC Guidelines for Field Triage of Injured Patients may appear highly technical. To simplify, it may be helpful to break the guidelines down into three distinct questions:

1. Does the patient have unstable vital signs and/or serious injuries that warrant transport to the highest-level trauma center?
2. Does the mechanism of injury warrant evaluation at a trauma center (not necessarily the highest level)?
3. Does the patient have extenuating circumstances that need to be considered for evaluation at a trauma center (not necessarily the highest level)?

Patients with concerning vital signs and/or apparent serious injuries warrant immediate stabilization and transport to the highest available trauma center in the region. In patients who have clinically stable vital signs, the presence of significant mechanism of injury may warrant evaluation at a trauma center, although it does not necessarily have to be the highest level available in the region. Patients who do not fall under the first two questions, but have extenuating circumstances (such as geriatric, pediatric, and pregnant patients, and patients with burns) may warrant consideration for trauma center evaluation. The best destination for these patients is based on their extenuating circumstances and consultation with medical control, if needed.

The CDC recommends that when in doubt, transport to a trauma center. It is better to overtriage rather than undertriage, although both should be avoided if possible.

Proper selection of which patients to transport to a trauma center involves a balance between "overtriage" and "undertriage." Overtriage and undertriage both result in worse outcomes for more critically injured patients because in overtriage resources can't keep up, and in undertriage the right resources aren't there. Transport decisions should also include compliance with local protocols or patient care map.

Balance Matters

To minimize undertriage, experts estimate that an overtriage rate of 30% to 50% is necessary, meaning that 30% to 50% of injured patients transported to a trauma center won't need the specialized care available there.

The commonly recognized definition for a "major trauma patient" is a patient with an Injury Severity Score (ISS) of 16 or higher.

ISS Assessment

Various scoring systems are used to analyze and categorize patients who suffer traumatic injury in the hospital setting. Scoring systems may also be used to predict patient outcomes based on the severity of their traumatic injury. These scoring systems generally are not calculated until the patient has been fully evaluated at the trauma center. They offer limited use in the initial triage of injured patients in the field, but they do have significant value in the overall quality assessment and quality improvement (QA/QI) process of trauma care delivery.

One of the most commonly discussed scoring systems is the Injury Severity Score (ISS). The ISS categorizes injuries into six anatomically distinct body regions:

1. Head and neck
2. Face
3. Chest
4. Abdomen
5. Extremities
6. External

Only the most severe injury in any one region is taken into account. After the most severe injuries in all six regions have been identified, they are assigned a value from 1 to 6 using the Abbreviated Injury Scale (AIS):

1. Minor
2. Moderate
3. Serious
4. Severe
5. Critical
6. Unsurvivable

The highest three values are then squared to give additional weight to the highest scores and minimize the lowest scores. These values are then added together to calculate the final ISS.

Higher ISS scores correlate linearly with mortality, morbidity, length of stay in the hospital, and other measures of severity. The major limitations of the ISS are that AIS scoring errors are amplified when calculated into the ISS, and there is no consideration given to the fact that injuries to certain areas of the body may inherently be more severe than injuries to other areas. While of limited use in the field triage of trauma patients, an understanding of how injury severity scores are calculated is highly valuable for the EMS provider when reading research articles and practice updates.

Unfortunately, you can't get a true ISS without advanced imaging, which isn't available in the field. In an effort to identify patients who would most benefit from a trauma center, the CDC published a report called "Guidelines for Field Triage of Injured Patients: Recommendations of the National Expert Panel."

These evidence-based guidelines assist EMS providers in making appropriate decisions about the transport destination of individual trauma patients.

The Field Triage Guidelines are broken down into four sections:

1. *Step I: Physiologic criteria.* This section includes:
   - Alteration in mental status (GCS < 14)
   - Hypotension (systolic blood pressure [SBP] < 90)
   - Respiratory abnormalities (ventilation rate [VR] < 10 or > 29 or need for ventilator support)
2. *Step II: Anatomic criteria.* If response times are short, patients may not have had a chance to develop significant physiological alterations even though they have life-threatening injuries. This section lists anatomic findings associated with severe injury.
3. *Step III: Mechanism of injury criteria.* These criteria identify additional patients who may have injuries that don't present with physiologic derangement or obvious external injury.
4. *Step IV: Special considerations.* These criteria identify how factors such as age, use of anticoagulants, or the presence of burns or pregnancy may affect the decision to transport to a trauma center.
   - Patients who meet either physiologic or anatomic injury criteria should be transported to the highest level of trauma care available.
   - Patients who meet mechanism of injury criteria should be transported to a trauma center but not necessarily to the highest level of trauma care.
   - Patients who meet the special considerations criteria may be transported to a trauma center or another capable hospital, based on clinical judgment and discussion with online medical control.

> **QUICK TIP**
> When in doubt, transport to a trauma center.

Duration of Transport

In simple terms, transport the patient to the closest appropriate facility (i.e., the closest facility most capable of managing the patient's problems). If the patient's injuries are severe or indicate continuing hemorrhage, you should take the patient to a facility that can provide definitive care as quickly as possible. Many nontrauma centers can't provide definitive care for severely injured patients and will transfer these patients to a trauma center.

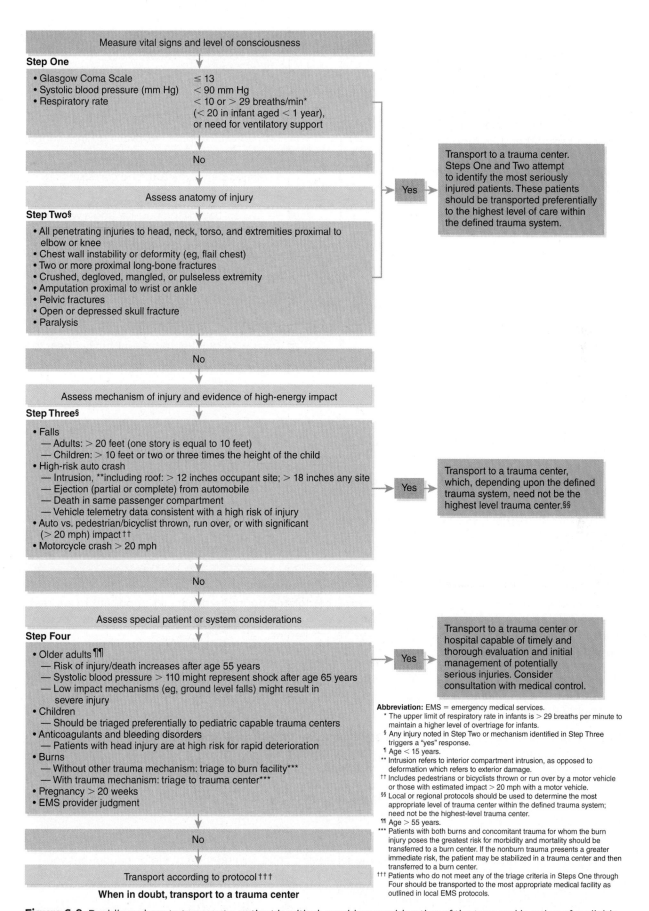

Measure vital signs and level of consciousness

Step One
- Glasgow Coma Scale ≤ 13
- Systolic blood pressure (mm Hg) < 90 mm Hg
- Respiratory rate < 10 or > 29 breaths/min*
  (< 20 in infant aged < 1 year),
  or need for ventilatory support

No

Assess anatomy of injury

Step Two§
- All penetrating injuries to head, neck, torso, and extremities proximal to elbow or knee
- Chest wall instability or deformity (eg, flail chest)
- Two or more proximal long-bone fractures
- Crushed, degloved, mangled, or pulseless extremity
- Amputation proximal to wrist or ankle
- Pelvic fractures
- Open or depressed skull fracture
- Paralysis

Yes → Transport to a trauma center. Steps One and Two attempt to identify the most seriously injured patients. These patients should be transported preferentially to the highest level of care within the defined trauma system.

No

Assess mechanism of injury and evidence of high-energy impact

Step Three§
- Falls
  — Adults: > 20 feet (one story is equal to 10 feet)
  — Children: > 10 feet or two or three times the height of the child
- High-risk auto crash
  — Intrusion, **including roof: > 12 inches occupant site; > 18 inches any site
  — Ejection (partial or complete) from automobile
  — Death in same passenger compartment
  — Vehicle telemetry data consistent with a high risk of injury
- Auto vs. pedestrian/bicyclist thrown, run over, or with significant (> 20 mph) impact††
- Motorcycle crash > 20 mph

Yes → Transport to a trauma center, which, depending upon the defined trauma system, need not be the highest level trauma center.§§

No

Assess special patient or system considerations

Step Four
- Older adults ¶¶
  — Risk of injury/death increases after age 55 years
  — Systolic blood pressure > 110 might represent shock after age 65 years
  — Low impact mechanisms (eg, ground level falls) might result in severe injury
- Children
  — Should be triaged preferentially to pediatric capable trauma centers
- Anticoagulants and bleeding disorders
  — Patients with head injury are at high risk for rapid deterioration
- Burns
  — Without other trauma mechanism: triage to burn facility***
  — With trauma mechanism: triage to trauma center***
- Pregnancy > 20 weeks
- EMS provider judgment

Yes → Transport to a trauma center or hospital capable of timely and thorough evaluation and initial management of potentially serious injuries. Consider consultation with medical control.

No

Transport according to protocol†††

When in doubt, transport to a trauma center

Abbreviation: EMS = emergency medical services.
  * The upper limit of respiratory rate in infants is > 29 breaths per minute to maintain a higher level of overtriage for infants.
  § Any injury noted in Step Two or mechanism identified in Step Three triggers a "yes" response.
  ¶ Age < 15 years.
  ** Intrusion refers to interior compartment intrusion, as opposed to deformation which refers to exterior damage.
  †† Includes pedestrians or bicyclists thrown or run over by a motor vehicle or those with estimated impact > 20 mph with a motor vehicle.
  §§ Local or regional protocols should be used to determine the most appropriate level of trauma center within the defined trauma system; need not be the highest-level trauma center.
  ¶¶ Age > 55 years.
  *** Patients with both burns and concomitant trauma for whom the burn injury poses the greatest risk for morbidity and mortality should be transferred to a burn center. If the nonburn trauma presents a greater immediate risk, the patient may be stabilized in a trauma center and then transferred to a burn center.
  ††† Patients who do not meet any of the triage criteria in Steps One through Four should be transported to the most appropriate medical facility as outlined in local EMS protocols.

Figure 6-8 Deciding where to transport a patient is critical, requiring consideration of the type and location of available facilities. Situations that will most likely require an in-house trauma team are detailed in the Field Triage Guidelines.

Modified from Centers for Disease Control and Prevention, *Morbidity and Mortality Weekly Report (MMWR)*, January 13, 2012.

The "How" Matters, Too

Some EMS systems have air transport available. Air medical services can offer a higher level of care than ground units for critically injured trauma victims. Air transport may also be quicker and smoother than ground transport in some circumstances. Helicopter EMS should be considered for those patients meeting guideline criteria for transport to the hospital with the highest level of care.

FOR MORE INFORMATION

Refer to the "Definitive Care in the Field" section of Chapter 6: Patient Assessment and Management.

PROGRESSIVE CASE STUDY: SUMMARY

- Secondary survey completed en route to hospital after primary survey completed on scene
- EMS unit transported to level II trauma center
- Patient was found to have a minimally displaced pelvic fracture and contusions to his upper back.
- He spent 4 days in the hospital and a week in rehab before going home for continued recovery.

Critical Actions:

- Pelvic binder
- Spinal motion restriction device
- Analgesia for pain management
- Cover with blanket to prevent further heat loss

LESSON WRAP-UP

- The secondary survey is a "search" for underlying injuries.
- Use the "see, hear, feel" approach for the secondary survey.
- Obtain "exact numbers" for your vital signs.
- Obtain a SAMPLE history.

PROGRESSIVE CASE STUDY RECAP

Part 1

For this patient, is the secondary survey performed in the field or during transport?	Secondary survey is completed during transport. It's important to address immediate life threats and quickly package this patient for transport to the appropriate trauma center.
What are the main objectives of the secondary survey?	A secondary head-to-toe evaluation of the patient to identify any injuries or problems not identified during the primary survey.
What is the importance of vital signs during the secondary survey?	■ Vital signs give you a quantitative evaluation of the patient's status. A complete set of vital signs includes: · Blood pressure (manual) · Pulse rate and quality · Ventilation rate and depth · Oxygen saturation · Skin color and temperature
What is the importance of the SAMPLE history during the secondary survey?	This mnemonic serves as a good reminder for the information that you should document for the patient care report and pass on to the medical staff at the receiving hospital.

How would you use "see, hear, feel" to complete the secondary survey?	■ See: • Be attentive for external or internal hemorrhage. • Examine all of the skin. • Note all soft-tissue injuries. • Note anything that does not "look right." ■ Hear • Note any unusual breathing sounds. • Note any abnormal sounds auscultated. • Verify whether breath sounds are present and equal. ■ Feel • Palpate all body regions. • Note any abnormal findings.
What types of clues can be "heard" during the secondary survey?	■ Adventitious lung sounds could lead you to unseen chest injuries. ■ A patient's inability to speak in full sentences, slurred speech, or asking repeated questions can lead you to head injury. ■ This patient speaks in full sentences and is alert and oriented. There is no slurring of or searching for words. ■ The patient continues to complain of lower and upper back pain that gets no better or worse with immobilization.
What could be "heard" that would indicate an injury to the neck?	■ Hoarseness in the voice could indicate a tracheal injury. ■ A bruit over the carotid artery can suggest a vascular injury. This patient has no hoarseness of the voice.
Could a patient's lung sounds lead you to hidden injuries?	Yes. Listen to the anterior and lateral chest of the immobilized patient. Remember to auscultate the lateral chest wall. Listen for diminished lung sounds, poor air movement, crackles, and crepitus.
When "feeling" for injuries on the head, what are your hands telling you?	Your hands will be able to find any lacerations, contusions, or deformities that may be hidden under the patient's hair. They'll also feel any instability in the bones of the face. This patient has none of these issues.
Can you assess ("feel") the patient's neck during the secondary survey?	The most sensitive area to palpate when clinically concerned for subcutaneous emphysema is above the sternum, along the patient's neck. It will be difficult with a cervical collar in place. If you can palpate the patient's neck, be aware of the presence of subcutaneous emphysema or crepitus of the trachea. This patient has a cervical collar in place, but his neck appears within normal limits during secondary survey.
How important is it to "feel" the patient's chest expand during the secondary survey?	Extremely important. By feeling the chest expand and contract during a deep breath, you can feel for crepitus, deformities, flail segments, paradoxical movement, or other abnormalities. It's especially important, because a patient with rib fractures will contract his/her muscles to splint his/her injury. This patient can take deep breaths, and his chest wall expands fully with some additional pain to his back. There are no abnormalities felt to the patient's chest wall.

(*continued*)

PROGRESSIVE CASE STUDY RECAP (*CONTINUED*)

Part 2

What injuries may be hidden in the abdomen? More importantly, what injuries may NOT be hidden in the abdomen?	■ Almost all injuries in the abdomen are hidden to prehospital care providers. The following injuries may be hidden: · Abdominal muscle injuries · Masses · Rigidity due to internal bleeding into the abdomen Remember to only palpate each quadrant once. This patient's abdomen is soft, nontender, and no masses found.
Why should palpation of the pelvis be done with caution?	Palpation of an unstable pelvis can cause bone fragments and clots to break loose, causing greater hemorrhage. You should look first and palpate the pelvis only once. When you apply gentle anterior-to-posterior pressure to this patient's pelvis, you notice instability.
What injuries might we find while "feeling" the extremities of this patient?	■ Crepitus ■ Pain ■ Tenderness ■ Unusual movements The extremities of this patient are found to be within normal limits.
When and how frequently should you calculate the patient's GCS?	The GCS of the patient should be assessed every time there's a change in the patient's condition and/or every time the patient's vital signs are assessed. This patient has a GCS of 15 when you arrive on scene and has a GCS of 15 throughout transport.
What can you tell from "looking into someone's eyes"?	By examining a patient's pupils, you'll be able to determine if there are any direct ocular injuries or if the patient has an underlying head injury caused by cerebral edema or an expanding intracranial hematoma. It's important to test a patient's sight (each eye separately). This patient's pupils are equal and reactive to light.
How often should you assess the patient's motor and sensory function?	Before and after immobilization of any kind and after moving the patient. This patient's motor and sensory function does not change throughout the scenario.

STUDY QUESTIONS

1. You arrive on the scene of a vehicle–pedestrian accident. The primary assessment reveals no immediate life-threatening injuries although the patient has an obvious deformity of her lower leg. What should you do?
   A. Conduct a detailed secondary survey.
   B. Conduct a focused secondary survey.
   C. Package the patient for transport to the nearest hospital.
   D. Get a SAMPLE history.

2. After assessing for life-threatening injuries, what should you do next?
   A. Obtain vital signs.
   B. Get a SAMPLE history.
   C. Conduct a head-to-toe physical examination.
   D. Treat the injuries.

3. How should you take a patient's blood pressure reading initially?
    A. With an automated, noninvasive blood pressure device
    B. Palpated
    C. Manually
    D. Pulse oximetry

4. At what point should you do a neurologic evaluation on the patient?
    A. At the very beginning of the secondary survey
    B. During your assessment of the head and face
    C. As the final step of the secondary survey
    D. Only when there is a clear change in mental status

5. The patient is in a lot of pain and is getting increasingly restless. What should you do?
    A. Nothing. The injury isn't life-threatening.
    B. Apply ice to the injury.
    C. Administer benzodiazepine.
    D. Administer an analgesic.

6. Why is it important to find out when a patient last ate when taking a SAMPLE history?
    A. It helps you determine whether any gastrointestinal issues are trauma related or not.
    B. Many trauma patients will require surgery, and recent food intake increases the risk of aspiration during induction of anesthesia.
    C. It helps determine what types of pain medication can and cannot be used.
    D. It determines the likelihood of whether the patient may vomit and aspirate.

7. Based on what you know, what is the patient's GCS?
    A. 15
    B. 12
    C. 10
    D. 8

ANSWER KEY

Question 1: A
The detailed physical examination is a head-to-toe examination that involves all areas of the body. The focused physical examination involves limited areas of the body. It is best in this circumstance to do a detailed assessment before packaging the patient for transport.

Question 2: A
After determining any life-threatening injuries, the next step is to obtain vital signs. After that you can get a SAMPLE history, conduct the physical examination and treat the injuries.

Question 3: C
Even if an automated, noninvasive blood pressure device is available, the initial blood pressure should be taken manually, since automated blood pressure devices may be inaccurate in patients in shock.

Question 4: C
You should begin at the head and proceed through the neck, chest, and abdomen to the extremities, concluding with a detailed neurologic examination.

Question 5: D
You can consider pain management in patients with isolated injuries, particularly in cases of prolonged transport, as long as signs of ventilatory impairment or shock aren't present. Sedation with an agent such as a benzodiazepine should only be used in exceptional circumstances—like a combative intubated patient.

Question 6: B
Many trauma patients will require surgery, and recent food intake increases the risk of aspiration during induction of anesthesia.

Question 7: A
The patient is alert and oriented, answers questions appropriately, and follows commands so her GCS is 15.

REFERENCES AND FURTHER READING

National Association of Emergency Medical Technicians. *PHTLS: Prehospital Trauma Life Support*. 9th ed. Burlington, MA: Public Safety Group; 2019.

Joint Trauma System. Pelvic Binders in TCCC. http://tccc.blubrry.net/2017/03/30/pelvic-binders-in-tccc/. Accessed November 13, 2018.

SKILL STATIONS

Pelvic Sling Application—Logrolling (Two Providers)*

1. Locate the greater trochanters.
2. Place the device under the patient by gently rolling the patient to one side, placing the device, and then rolling the patient back.
3. Feed the black precision strap through the buckle.
4. Your partner pulls the black strap with one hand while the second pulls the orange handle in the opposite direction.
5. Pull until an audible click is heard and felt at the buckle. Note: If using the SAM Pelvic Sling, do not be concerned if a second click is heard after the sling is secured.
6. Maintain traction on the black strap and the orange handle while securing the strap onto itself.

Pelvic Sling Application Alternative—Lifting (Two Providers)

1. Locate the greater trochanters.
2. Gently lift the patient and slide the device under the patient's pelvis.
3. Feed the black precision strap through the buckle.
4. Pull the black strap while your partner pulls the orange handle in the opposite direction.
5. Pull until an audible click is heard and felt at the buckle. Note: If using the SAM Pelvic Sling, do not be concerned if a second click is heard after the sling secured.
6. While maintaining traction, the strap is secured onto itself.

*SAM Pelvic sling instructions from: http://www.sammedical.com/assets/uploads/SLI-PED-G-01_FEB-2018-STATIC-sm.pdf

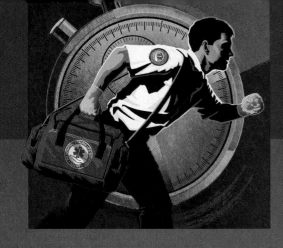

Disability: Traumatic Brain Injury

LESSON OBJECTIVES

- Identify the signs and symptoms of traumatic brain injury (TBI).
- Explain the pathophysiology of TBI.
- Discuss the biomechanics of injury that cause TBI.
- Distinguish primary and secondary brain injuries.
- Demonstrate proper medical management of traumatic brain injuries.

Introduction

Traumatic brain injury (TBI) is a worldwide public health problem that affects over 10 million people annually across the globe. According to the World Health Organization (WHO), TBI will surpass many diseases as the major cause of death and disability by 2020.

That's a Lot of Headaches

In the United States, approximately 2.8 million TBI-related events occur yearly, including deaths, hospitalizations, and emergency department (ED) visits. This total equates to one person sustaining a TBI every 21 seconds.

TBI is the most frequent cause of death and disability among children in the United States, with more than a million children sustaining brain injuries yearly. Over 80% of all TBIs are mild, but approximately 282,000 patients are hospitalized, and each year 50,000 die from moderate to severe TBIs.

Common causes of TBIs include:

- Motor vehicle collisions
- Falls
- Violence
- Workplace or sports-related unintentional injuries

Crashes and Falls

Motor vehicle crashes are the leading cause of TBI in patients between the ages of 5 and 75 years of age, while falls are the leading cause of TBI in pediatric patients up to 4 years of age and in the older adult population.

Patients with TBI can be some of the most challenging trauma patients to treat. They may be combative and attempts to manage the airway can be difficult because of clenched jaw muscles and vomiting. Assessment can be further hindered by shock from other injuries or drug and/or alcohol intoxication. Occasionally serious intracranial injuries are present, but there is minimal or no external evidence of trauma.

Skilled care in the prehospital setting focuses on ensuring the adequate delivery of oxygen and nutrients to the brain and rapidly identifying patients at risk for herniation and elevated intracranial pressure. This approach decreases mortality and reduces the incidence of permanent neurologic disability. Our goal when treating TBI is to keep further harm from occurring to even a single brain cell and to establish conditions optimal for healing and recovery.

PROGRESSIVE CASE STUDY: PART 1

PROGRESSIVE CASE STUDY: PART 1

You are dispatched to a report of a male who was riding at a skatepark, fell, and hit his head. When you arrive, you observe the area and discover a small group of boys and young men standing around the patient. There are no safety hazards at this point.

The patient is 22 years old. His friend tells you they were trying to see who could ride the longest down the rail when his skateboard went out from underneath him and he fell. He put his hand out to stop himself, struck his hand first, and then fell, striking his head on the concrete.

The patient was not wearing a helmet. He is currently lying prone on the ground and has a hematoma and abrasions to the right side of the head near the top.

Questions:

- What are the concerning physics of trauma for this patient?
- What injuries may the patient have incurred?

FOR MORE INFORMATION

Refer to the "Anatomy" section of Chapter 8: Head Trauma.

Physiology Review
Cerebral Blood Flow

It's critical that the brain's neurons receive a constant flow of blood so they can provide oxygen and glucose. This constant cerebral blood flow is maintained by ensuring:

1. An adequate pressure (cerebral perfusion pressure) to force blood through the brain
2. A regulatory mechanism (autoregulation) that ensures constant blood flow by varying the resistance to blood flow as the perfusion pressure changes.

Cerebral Perfusion Pressure

Cerebral perfusion pressure is the amount of pressure available to push blood through the cerebral circulation and maintain blood flow and oxygen and glucose delivery to the energy-demanding cells of the brain. Cerebral perfusion pressure relates directly to the patient's mean arterial pressure (MAP) and ICP. The MAP is the average pressure in the arteries during one cardiac cycle and is an indicator of perfusion to vital organs.

Cerebral perfusion pressure is expressed by the following formula:

$$\text{Cerebral perfusion pressure} = \text{Mean arterial pressure} - \text{Intracranial pressure}$$

or

$$CPP = MAP - ICP$$

MAP Those Numbers

Normal MAP ranges from 85 to 95 mm Hg. In adults, ICP is normally below 15 mm Hg. It's usually 3 to 7 mm Hg in children and 1.5 to 6 mm Hg in infants. Therefore, cerebral perfusion pressure is normally about 70 to 80 mm Hg. Sudden increases or decreases in blood pressure and ICP may affect cerebral perfusion.

Autoregulation of Cerebral Blood Flow

The most important factor for the brain isn't cerebral perfusion pressure but rather cerebral blood flow. The brain works very hard at keeping its blood flow constant over a wide range of changing conditions. This process is known as autoregulation. Autoregulation is crucial to the brain's normal function.

To understand autoregulation, we need to remember that for any flowing system:

$$\text{Pressure} = \text{Flow} \times \text{Resistance}$$

In the case of the brain, this translates into:

$$\text{Cerebral perfusion pressure} = \text{Cerebral blood flow} \times \text{Cerebral vascular resistance}$$

or

$$CPP = CBF \times CVR$$

Because the brain's principal concern is cerebral blood flow, it's useful to rewrite this equation as:

$$CBF = CPP/CVR$$

If cerebral perfusion pressure decreases, the only way to keep blood flow constant is by decreasing vascular resistance. The brain accomplishes autoregulation by adjusting cerebral vascular resistance (through vasodilation), but this mechanism requires a certain minimum cerebral perfusion pressure. Below a cerebral perfusion pressure of about 50 mm Hg, the autoregulatory mechanisms can no longer compensate for the decreased cerebral perfusion pressure, and cerebral blood flow starts to decrease.

> ### QUICK TIP
>
> At a pressure of 0 mm Hg, no amount of vasodilation will cause blood to flow, and there are limits to how much the blood vessels in the head can dilate.

In the face of reduced cerebral blood flow, the brain tissues will extract more oxygen from the blood. However, once the oxygen extraction limit is met, mental status will begin to deteriorate.

If ICP increases due to bleeding or trauma, more pressure will be needed to force blood flow across the brain. If the needed pressure is not attained, ischemic brain damage will occur.

The relationship between cerebral perfusion pressure, ICP, and MAP is important in trauma. Acute intracranial bleeding causes compression to surrounding tissues and an increased ICP. This is termed mass effect. As the ICP increases, the amount of pressure needed to push blood through the brain also increases. The MAP will increase to maintain CPP. If the MAP can't keep up with the increase in ICP or if treatment to decrease the ICP isn't started quickly, the amount of blood flowing through the brain decreases, leading to ischemic brain damage and impaired brain function. In the absence of an ICP monitor, the best practice is to maintain a high-normal MAP.

> ### QUICK TIP
>
> The Brain Trauma Foundation recommends maintaining systolic blood pressure greater than 90 mm Hg for neurologically injured patients.

Oxygen and Cerebral Blood Flow

The brain has high oxygen requirements. Decreased levels of oxygen (hypoxia) cause major vasodilation in an effort to increase cerebral blood flow. This response typically doesn't occur until the arterial oxygen partial pressure (Pao_2) falls below 50 mm Hg, but when it does, it can further increase brain volume and therefore intracranial pressure.

Carbon Dioxide and Cerebral Blood Flow

The cerebral blood vessels respond to changes in arterial carbon dioxide levels by either constricting or dilating. Decreased levels of carbon dioxide (hypocapnia) result in vasoconstriction, while elevated levels (hypercapnia) cause vasodilation.

Hyperventilation reduces the $Paco_2$ by increasing the rate at which carbon dioxide gets blown off by the lungs. The resulting hypocapnia changes the acid–base balance in the brain, resulting in vasoconstriction. This reduces the intravascular volume of the brain, reducing cerebral blood volume and, therefore, often ICP. However, this comes at a price, which is reduced cerebral perfusion.

> **Hyperventilation, Blood Flow, and ICP**
>
> Hyperventilation has been used to reduce ICP but also adversely impacts cerebral blood flow. In fact, data suggest that hyperventilation more reliably reduces cerebral blood flow than ICP.

> ### CASE STUDY PROGRESSION: PART 2
>
> Your primary survey reveals the following:
>
> - **X**—Oozing of dark blood from the right side of the head
> - **A**—Patent, you see no airway obstruction; your partner is performing manual in-line stabilization.
> - **B**—Breathing is increased, 20 breaths/min, lungs clear bilaterally.
> - **C**—Skin is pale, warm, and dry; pulse 100 beats/min, Spo_2 92%, $ETco_2$ 32 mm Hg.
> - **D**—Patient is conscious, confused, GCS 13 (E3, V4, M6), pupils 3 mm and equal bilaterally; you notice an open fracture of the distal right radius/ulna. No active exsanguination
> - **E**—Outside temp is warm 78°F (25°C). Patient's skin temp is normal. Right forearm is deformed with a bleeding open fracture.
>
> **Questions:**
> - Is there a need for hemorrhage control?
> - Is airway management indicated?
> - Is spinal motion restriction indicated?
> - Could this patient have a traumatic brain injury?

CRITICAL-THINKING QUESTIONS

Why is airway management important in a patient with TBI?

Hypoxia is a major concern with a TBI. Irreversible brain damage can occur after only 4 to 6 minutes of arterial desaturation in the injured brain. A significant number of TBI patients present with low or inadequate SpO_2, which may be missed without use of pulse oximetry.

You must ensure adequate circulation by minimizing blood loss and adequate oxygenation by maintaining a patent airway and adequate ventilation.

Does oxygen saturation or ETCO₂ tell us more about the ventilatory status of a patient with TBI?

Remember that a ventilatory rate between 10 to 20 breaths/min in an adult TBI patient and an oxygen saturation rate of 94% or greater are the most important. $ETCO_2$ isn't always reliable in an unstable patient and only provides a rough estimate of hypoventilation or hyperventilation in the TBI patient; however, you should try to maintain an $ETCO_2$ between 35 to 40 mm Hg for a TBI patient.

FOR MORE INFORMATION

Refer to the "Physiology" section of Chapter 8: Head Trauma.

Pathophysiology of Primary Brain Injury

TBI can be divided into two categories: primary and secondary. Primary brain injury occurs at the time of the original insult and is any injury that occurs due to the initial trauma. This includes injury to the brain, its coverings, and associated vascular structures.

Primary brain injuries include:

- Brain contusions
- Hemorrhages
- Damage to nerves and brain vessels

Because neural tissue doesn't regenerate well and because it can't really be repaired, there won't be much recovery of the structure and function lost due to primary injury.

Cerebral Concussion

The diagnosis of a "concussion" is made as a result of the presence of symptoms persisting after mild TBI. Most people associate a loss of consciousness with the diagnosis of concussion, but it's not required to make the diagnosis.

I Don't Remember

The hallmark of concussion is actually posttraumatic amnesia, a state of confusion following trauma where the patient is disoriented and unable to recall events that occurred before (retrograde) and after (anterograde) injury. These patients may become agitated because they don't understand or recall what's going on.

Table 7A-1 Cantu Concussion Grading System	
Severity	**Description**
Grade 1: Mild	No loss of consciousness
	Posttraumatic amnesia or postconcussion signs or symptoms lasting less than 30 minutes
Grade 2: Moderate	Loss of consciousness lasting less than 1 minute
	Posttraumatic amnesia or postconcussion signs or symptoms lasting longer than 30 minutes but less than 24 hours
Grade 3: Severe	Loss of consciousness lasting more than 1 minute
	Posttraumatic amnesia lasting more than 24 hours; postconcussion signs or symptoms lasting longer than 7 days

© Jones & Bartlett Learning.

Other neurologic changes include:

- Vacant stare (befuddled facial expression)
- Delayed verbal and motor responses (slow to answer questions or follow instructions)

- Confusion and inability to focus attention (easily distracted and unable to follow through with normal activities)
- Disorientation (walking in the wrong direction; unaware of time, date, and place)
- Slurred or incoherent speech (making disjointed or incomprehensible statements)
- Lack of coordination (stumbling, inability to walk tandem/straight line)
- Emotions inappropriate to the circumstances (distraught, crying for no apparent reason)
- Memory deficits (exhibited by patient repeatedly asking the same question that has already been answered)
- Inability to memorize and recall (e.g., three out of three words or three out of three objects in 5 minutes)

It's Not the Flu

Over the past few years, the medical community has recognized the significance of the long-term impact of cerebral concussion. Severe headache, dizziness, nausea, and vomiting frequently accompany a concussion. Patients exhibiting signs of concussion, especially patients with nausea, vomiting, or neurologic findings on secondary survey, should be immediately transported for further evaluation. The formal diagnosis of a concussion will be made in the hospital once the patient has been evaluated and a head CT scan result shows no observable intracranial pathology. Concussion requires a thorough follow-up, as the symptoms and the susceptibility to secondary injury can last for weeks.

Diffuse Axonal Injury (DAI)

Diffuse axonal injury (DAI) is widespread damage to the nerve axons. This happens because of shearing injury to the nerve cells (gray-white matter) due to rapid acceleration or deceleration (car accidents, falls, blows to the head), especially in the brain stem. The main symptom associated with DIA is persistent coma in spite of minimal radiologic signs on CT scan.

There is currently no definitive treatment for this injury beyond normal head injury protocol with a focus on reducing the ICP.

Intracranial Hematoma

Intracranial hematomas are divided into four general types:

- Epidural
- Subdural
- Subarachnoid
- Intracerebral

Because the signs and symptoms of each have definite overlap, specific diagnosis in the prehospital setting (as well as the ED) is almost impossible. You may suspect a particular type of hematoma based on the characteristic clinical presentation, but a definitive diagnosis can be made only after a CT scan. Because these hematomas occupy space inside the rigid skull, they may produce rapid increases in ICP, especially if they're sizable.

Epidural Hematoma

Epidural hematomas often result from a low-velocity blow to the temporal bone, such as the impact from a punch or baseball. A fracture of this thin bone damages the middle meningeal artery, which results in arterial bleeding that collects between the skull and dura mater. This high-pressure arterial blood can start to dissect, or peel, the dura off of the inner table of the skull, creating an epidural space full of blood. The principal threat to the brain is from the expanding mass of blood displacing the brain and threatening herniation.

The classic sign for an epidural hematoma is a patient experiencing a brief loss of consciousness, then regaining consciousness, and then experiencing a rapid decline in consciousness. During the period of consciousness (the lucid interval) the patient may be oriented, lethargic, or confused or may complain of a headache. A patient who experiences a "lucid interval," followed by a decline in GCS score, needs emergency evaluation. As a patient's consciousness worsens, the physical examination may reveal a dilated and sluggish or nonreactive pupil, most commonly on the ipsilateral (same) side of the herniation.

Subdural Hematoma

In addition to being more common than epidural hematomas, subdural hematomas differ in etiology, location, and prognosis. Unlike the epidural hematoma, which is caused by arterial hemorrhage, a subdural hematoma generally results from a venous bleed and is associated with direct brain injury. In this case, bridging veins are torn during a violent blow to the head. Blood collects in the subdural space, between the dura mater and the underlying arachnoid membrane.

Subdural hematomas present in two different ways:

1. In patients who've experienced significant trauma, the tearing of the bridging veins results in a rapid accumulation of blood in the subdural space, with rapid onset of mass effect. These patients will exhibit an acutely depressed mental status and will need immediate transport to

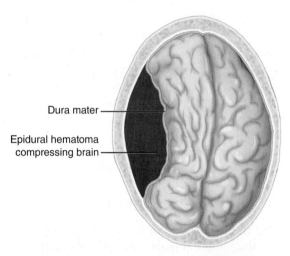

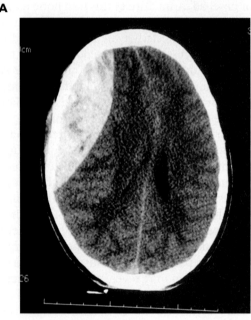

Figure 7A-1 A. Epidural hematoma. **B.** CT scan of epidural hematoma.

A: © National Association of Emergency Medical Technicians. B: Courtesy of Peter T. Pons, MD, FACEP.

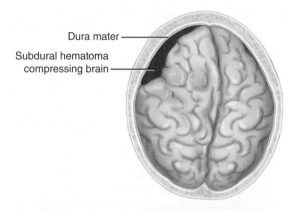

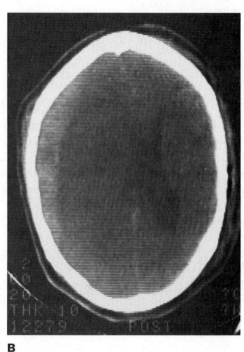

Figure 7A-2 A. Subdural hematoma. **B.** CT scan of subdural hematoma.

A: © National Association of Emergency Medical Technicians. B: Courtesy of Peter T. Pons, MD, FACEP.

an appropriate receiving facility for CT scan, ICP monitoring and management, and possibly surgery.

2. Clinically occult subdural hematomas can also occur. In older adults or patients with chronic diseases, the subdural space enlarges due to

---

It's Not the Height of the Fall That Counts

Older patients receiving anticoagulants such as warfarin (Coumadin) are at higher risk. Because these falls are minor, patients often don't get evaluated and the bleeds aren't identified.

---

brain atrophy. Blood may accumulate in the subdural space without causing mass effect and can remain asymptomatic for a long time. Such subdural hematomas can occur during falls in older adults or during minor trauma.

Because the onset of the mass effect is gradual, the patient doesn't have the dramatic signs associated with an acute subdural hematoma. Instead, the patient is more likely to present with headache, visual disturbances, personality changes, difficulty speaking (dysarthria), and hemiparesis or hemiplegia that is slow to progress. A chronic subdural hematoma might only be discovered when some of these symptoms become obvious enough to prompt the patient or caregiver to seek help.

Older Noggin, Greater Risk

In the geriatric patient:

- Veins are more susceptible to tearing, increasing the risk of a subdural hematoma from minor blunt trauma.
- Brain atrophy results in increased space in the cranial vault.
- A larger volume of blood may accumulate before outward signs of increased intracranial pressure are present.

Subarachnoid Hemorrhage

Subarachnoid hemorrhage (SAH) is bleeding that occurs under the arachnoid membrane. Blood in the subarachnoid space can't enter the subdural space. Many of the brain's blood vessels are located in the subarachnoid space, so injury to these vessels causes subarachnoid bleeding, a layering of blood beneath the arachnoid membrane on the surface of the brain. This is typically thin and rarely causes mass effect.

SAH usually results from a spontaneous rupture of cerebral aneurysms and causes the sudden onset of the worst headache of the patient's life. Patients usually complain of headaches, which may be severe, as well as nausea, vomiting, and dizziness. In addition, the presence of blood in the subarachnoid space can cause meningeal signs like pain and stiffness of the neck, visual complaints, and photophobia (aversion to bright light).

Follow My Finger

Bleeding from the posterior communicating artery can cause oculomotor nerve abnormalities or loss of movement on the ipsilateral (same) side; the affected eye will look down and outward, and patients can't lift their eyelids. These patients may also develop seizures, although seizure development is more common in cerebral aneurysm rupture or arteriovenous malformations.

PROGRESSIVE CASE STUDY: PART 3

Questions:

- Is airway management necessary for your patient?
- What does the patient's ETCO$_2$ tell you about him?
- How would you manage this patient's initial oxygen needs?
- Is spinal motion restriction indicated?

Intracranial Hematomas

Damage to the brain itself may produce cerebral contusions. If the damage includes injury to the blood vessels in the brain, there will be bleeding within the brain, known as intracerebral hematomas. Cerebral contusions are common both in patients with severe brain injuries and in those with moderate head injuries. Contusions often occur in locations far from the site of impact, often on the opposite side of the brain (coup-contrecoup injury).

Cerebral contusions often take 12 to 24 hours to appear on CT scans. The only clue to its presence may be a depressed GCS score. These contusions can increase dramatically in patients taking anticoagulants or antiplatelets.

Skull Fractures

Skull fractures can result from either blunt or penetrating trauma. Linear fractures are usually from blunt trauma. However, a powerful impact may produce a depressed skull fracture, where fragments of bone are driven toward or into the underlying brain tissue.

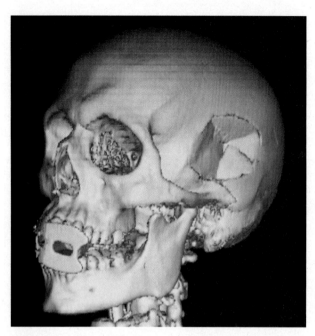

Figure 7A-3 A three-dimensional reconstruction of a depressed skull fracture after an assault.
Courtesy of Peter T. Pons, MD, FACEP.

Although the only way to diagnose simple linear fractures is with radiography, you may be able to feel a depressed skull fracture during a careful physical examination.

Here are a few of things to keep in mind:

- A closed, nondepressed skull fracture by itself doesn't mean much, but its presence increases the risk of an intracranial hematoma.
- Closed, depressed skull fractures may require neurosurgical intervention because the decrease in intracranial space by the encroaching fracture results in increased ICP and an underlying cerebral injury is often present.
- Open skull fractures can happen during a particularly forceful impact or a gunshot wound and serve as an entry site for bacteria, predisposing the patient to meningitis. If the dura mater is torn, brain tissue or CSF may leak from an open skull fracture. Because of the risk of meningitis, these wounds require immediate neurosurgical evaluation.

Basilar Skull Fractures

Basilar skull fractures are fractures of the base of the skull that most commonly involve temporal bone fractures. These fractures can cause tears in membranes, resulting in CSF leakage. In approximately 12% to 30% of basilar skull fractures, CSF can leak from the ears through a perforated eardrum (otorrhea) or from the nostrils (rhinorrhea).

Periorbital ecchymosis ("raccoon eyes") and Battle's sign, where bruising appears over the mastoid area behind the ears, can occur with basilar skull fractures, although they may take several hours after injury to become apparent.

> **QUICK TIP**
>
> Examination of the tympanic membrane with an otoscope may reveal blood behind the eardrum, indicating a basilar skull fracture.

> **FOR MORE INFORMATION**
>
> *Refer to the "Specific Head and Neck" section of Chapter 8: Head Trauma.*

Secondary Brain Injury

Injured brain tissue is extremely susceptible to further injury, and many secondary injuries can lead to the death of brain cells that would have otherwise survived. The most devastating secondary injuries are second impact (important in soft injuries), hypoxia, and hypotension. Secondary brain injury is continued injury or injury to structures that were originally injured but not destroyed by the primary brain injury. Once an injury occurs, a number of processes kick in, making the brain vulnerable to further injury for hours to even weeks after the initial insult. The main goal in the management of TBI is to identify and limit or stop these secondary injury mechanisms.

> **The Hidden Villain**
>
> The secondary effects are insidious and there's often significant, ongoing damage that isn't immediately apparent. These effects play a major role in death and disability after TBIs. By understanding what type of secondary injury is likely to occur as a result of the primary trauma, we can prepare for and intervene to correct or prevent these complications from occurring.

Mechanisms related to intracranial mass effect, elevated ICP, and mechanical shifting of the brain can lead to herniation and need to be addressed quickly. Management has been revolutionized by computed tomography (CT) scanning and other advanced imaging equipment, ICP monitoring, and immediate surgery.

Two other important causes of secondary injury are hypoxia and hypotension. Unrecognized and untreated hypoxia and hypotension are as harmful to the injured brain as elevated ICP. In addition, impaired oxygen or glucose delivery to an injured brain is more devastating than in the normal brain. Therefore, it's critical to avoid and/or treat hypoxia and hypotension as much as possible.

Mass Effect and Herniation

The secondary injury mechanisms you'll see most often are those related to mass effect. They're the result of the complex interactions between the brain, CSF, and blood against the skull, described by the Monro-Kellie doctrine. This doctrine states that the sum of the volume of brain tissue, blood, and CSF must remain constant with an intact skull. An increase in one component (such as from a hematoma, cerebral swelling, or tumor) causes a decrease in one or two of the other components or the ICP will increase.

In response to an expanding mass, the brain's first compensatory mechanism is to decrease the volume of intracranial CSF. The CSF circulates within and around the brain, brain stem, and spinal cord, but as the mass expands, CSF gets forced out of the head. Venous drainage also increases to help reduce blood volume inside the cranial vault. These two mechanisms prevent ICP from rising during the early phase of mass accumulation, and the patient may seem asymptomatic. As the mass size increases past the threshold of blood and CSF removal, ICP will start to increase rapidly. The effect of the mass is to shift the brain across and through fixed structures in the skull, eventually causing portions of the brain to herniate through or around some of them. This causes compression of the brain's most vital centers and jeopardizes their arterial blood supply.

The consequences of this movement toward and through the foramen magnum are described as the

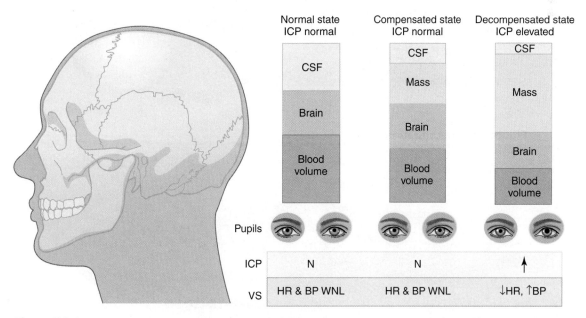

Figure 7A-4 Monro-Kellie doctrine: The volume of intracranial contents must remain constant. If the addition of a mass such as a hematoma results in the decrease of an equal volume of CSF and blood, the ICP remains normal. However, when this compensatory mechanism is exhausted, an exponential increase in ICP occurs for minute increases in the volume of the hematoma.

various herniation syndromes. These syndromes can occur in combination with each other.

Clinical Herniation Syndromes

Certain features of the syndromes can help identify a patient who is herniating. In uncal herniation:

- Compression of CN III results in a dilated or blown pupil on the same side of the herniation.
- Loss of function of the motor tract results in weakness on the opposite (contralateral) side of the body and the Babinski reflex.
- More extensive herniation can result in destruction of the red nucleus or the vestibular nuclei in the brain stem. This can result in decorticate posturing, which involves abnormal flexion of the upper extremities and rigidity and extension of the lower extremities.
- A more ominous finding is decerebrate posturing, in which all extremities extend and arching of the spine may occur. Decerebrate posturing occurs with injury and damage to the brain stem.

It Gets Worse

Herniation may lead to a terminal event where the extremities become flaccid, and motor activity is absent.

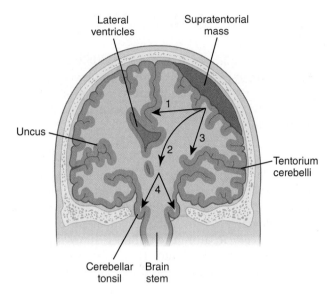

Figure 7A-5 The various herniation syndromes that can result from mass effect and increased ICP: (1) cingulate herniation, (2) central herniation, (3) uncal herniation, (4) cerebellotonsillar herniation. These syndromes can occur in combination with each other.

© Jones & Bartlett Learning.

As herniation progresses to central and tonsillar herniation, it affects the reticular activating system, causing abnormal ventilatory patterns or apnea, with

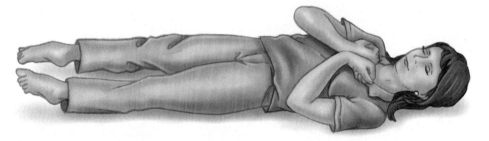

Figure 7A-6 Decorticate posturing.

© Jones & Bartlett Learning.

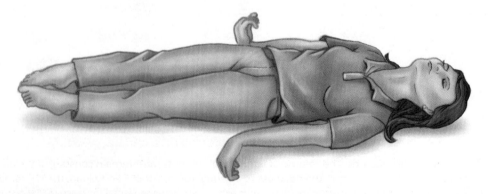

Figure 7A-7 Decerebrate posturing.

© Jones & Bartlett Learning.

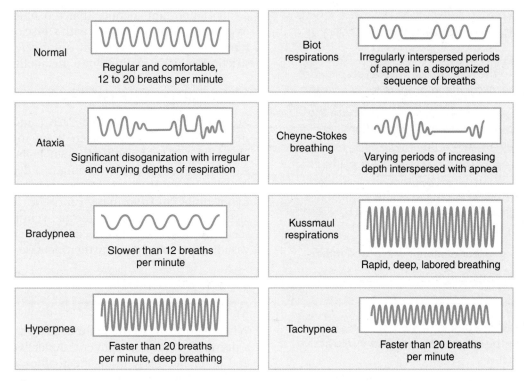

Figure 7A-8 This image demonstrates the various types of breathing patterns that may occur after head and brain trauma.

Modified from *Mosby's Guide to Physical Examination*, Seidel HM, Ball JW, Dains JE, et al. Copyright Elsevier (Mosby), 1999.

worsening hypoxia and significantly altered blood carbon dioxide levels.

To battle rising ICP, the autonomic nervous system kicks in to increase systemic blood pressure (and MAP) to maintain a normal cerebral perfusion pressure. Systolic pressures can reach up to 250 mm Hg. But as the baroreceptors in the carotid arteries and aortic arch sense the greatly increased blood pressure, messages are shot off to the brain stem to activate the parasympathetic nervous system. A signal then travels via the 10th cranial nerve, the vagus nerve, to slow the heart rate.

Cushing Phenomenon

Cushing phenomenon describes the combination of findings that occur with increased ICP: bradycardia, increased blood pressure associated with a widened pulse pressure, and irregular respirations, such as Cheyne-Stokes breathing.

Hypotension

Brain ischemia is common in severe brain injury. Studies have identified it in 90% of patients who die of TBI, and in many survivors. Therefore, the impact of low cerebral blood flow on TBI outcomes is a primary focus for limiting secondary injury after TBI.

In the national TBI database, the two most significant predictors of poor outcome from TBI were:

- The amount of time spent with an ICP greater than 20 mm Hg
- The time spent with a systolic blood pressure less than 90 mm Hg

Several studies have confirmed the profound impact of low systolic blood pressure on the outcome after TBI.

QUICK TIP

Many patients with TBI sustain other injuries, often involving bleeding and subsequent hypotension. Fluid resuscitation, as well as rapid definitive treatment of these injuries, intended to maintain systolic blood pressure of at least 90 mm Hg is essential to limit secondary injury to the brain.

Hypoxia and Hyperoxia

Irreversible brain damage can occur after only 4 to 6 minutes of cerebral anoxia (oxygen starvation to the brain). An oxygen saturation of hemoglobin (SpO_2) less than 90% in TBI patients will have a profound negative impact. Adequate ventilation and blood flow are critical in maintaining adequate oxygen delivery to the brain.

PROGRESSIVE CASE STUDY: PART 4

You apply spinal motion restriction and move the patient to the ambulance where you provide supplemental oxygen and prepare for IV access.

As you start your secondary survey, you note the patient is no longer talking to you. Secondary survey reveals the following:

- HEENT—Patient has a laceration in the right temporal region with a depression of the skull. Pupils—left 3 mm, right 5 mm and nonreactive. Neck—no step off or pain was noted when cervical collar applied.

- Chest—Lungs clear bilaterally, no noted injury

- Abdomen—Soft, nontender, no masses

- Pelvis—Intact

- Extremities/neurologic—Patient has an open fracture of the distal right radius/ulna. No active exsanguination.

Vital Signs:

- BP: 168/112 mm Hg

- Heart rate and quality: 56 beats/min at radial

- Ventilation rate: 10 breaths/min, irregular rate and depth

- SpO_2: 90%/RA

- $ETCO_2$: 48 mm Hg

- GCS: 4 (E1, V1, M2)

- Glucose: 110 mg/dl (6.1 mmol/l)

- Skin condition and temperature: Pale skin

- Temperature: 101°F (38.4°C)

- Pain: Unable to assess

Questions:

- What is the appropriate IV access this patient should receive?

- What do the unequal pupils indicate in this patient?

- What is most likely happening in the brain cavity?

- What type of injury could be causing the patient to be unconscious?

It's important to note that too much oxygen, or hyperoxia, is also associated with worse outcomes. One hundred percent oxygen can cause cerebral vasoconstriction, which can alter brain metabolism.

Hypocapnia and Hypercapnia

Both hypocapnia (decreased $Paco_2$) and hypercapnia (increased $Paco_2$) can worsen brain injury. Cerebral blood flow is compromised when blood vessels constrict due to hypocapnia, leading to a decrease in oxygen delivery to the brain. Hypercapnia is the result of hypoventilation from many causes, including drug or alcohol intoxication and abnormal ventilation patterns seen in patients with increased ICP. Hypercapnia causes vasodilation, which can further increase ICP.

Hypoglycemia and Hyperglycemia

When blood flow to the brain decreases, in addition to a decrease in oxygen delivery, the delivery of glucose and other necessary brain metabolites also decreases. Glucose is the primary fuel source of the adult brain, and changes in cerebral glucose metabolism are a common response to TBI. Both elevations (hyperglycemia) and decreases (hypoglycemia) in blood glucose can jeopardize ischemic brain tissue.

QUICK TIP

Elevated blood glucose levels have been associated with poorer neurologic outcome and should be avoided.

In the prehospital environment, the emphasis should be on avoiding hypoglycemia because the physiologic threat from low glucose is much more immediate than the danger from elevated serum glucose. Perform blood glucose measurement in all patients with altered mental status and, if found to be below normal values, administer glucose.

Too Much Is Better Than Too Little

Any induced hyperglycemia is likely to be transient, and the tight glucose control required to manage these patients properly will be established upon admission to the hospital.

Seizures

A patient with acute TBI is at risk for seizures for several reasons:

- Hypoxia from airway or breathing problems can cause generalized seizure activity, as can hypoglycemia and electrolyte abnormalities.
- Ischemic or damaged brain tissue can produce grand mal seizures or status epilepticus.
- Seizures can aggravate preexisting hypoxia.
- Seizures can further harm the injured brain because the neuronal activity associated with generalized seizures rapidly depletes oxygen and glucose levels, which further worsens cerebral ischemia.

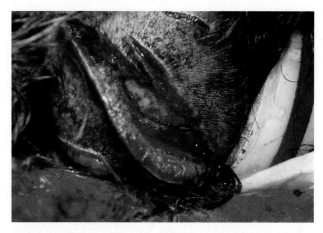

Figure 7A-9 Extensive scalp injuries may result in massive external hemorrhage.
Courtesy of Peter T. Pons, MD, FACEP.

PROGRESSIVE CASE STUDY: PART 5

Questions:

- How would you prevent secondary brain injury for the patient in this case?
- What injuries does the patient have that may precipitate secondary brain injury?

FOR MORE INFORMATION

Refer to the "Physiology" section of Chapter 8: Head Trauma.

Primary Survey

Exsanguinating Hemorrhage

The scalp has multiple layers of tissue and is highly vascular. Injuries to this area vary from simple small lacerations to complex injuries like a degloving injury, where a large area of the scalp gets torn back from the skull.

Uncontrolled hemorrhage from these injuries can result in hypovolemic shock and even exsanguination. This type of injury often occurs in an unrestrained front-seat occupant of a vehicle whose head impacts the windshield, as well as in workers whose long hair becomes caught in machinery. A serious blow to the head may result in the formation of a scalp hematoma, which may be confused with a depressed skull fracture while palpating the scalp.

Airway & Breathing

TBI causes loss of consciousness, which makes the patient less able to maintain and protect his or her airway. Emesis, hemorrhage, and swelling from facial trauma are common causes of airway difficulty in patients with TBI. Adequate oxygen delivery to the injured brain is essential to minimize secondary brain injury. Maintaining Spo_2 above 90% is critical.

Several different breathing patterns can result from severe brain injury, especially if the brain stem is involved or if intracranial pressure is increased. That is why assisted ventilation can become necessary in severe TBI cases.

Circulation

Maintaining a systolic blood pressure greater than 90 mm Hg is also critical in the prevention of secondary brain injury, so control any bleeding fast to prevent and/or minimize hypotension. Uncontrolled bleeding from a scalp injury can be an unrecognized cause of hemorrhagic shock and should be controlled as quickly as possible with direct pressure or a pressure dressing.

If possible, also note any external bleeding and the amount of blood present.

In the absence of significant external blood loss, a weak, rapid pulse in a victim of blunt trauma suggests life-threatening internal hemorrhage in the pleural spaces, peritoneum, retroperitoneum, or soft tissues surrounding long-bone fractures. In an infant with open fontanelles, sufficient blood loss can occur inside the cranium to bring on hypovolemic shock.

Disability

After you've started treatment for problems identified during the primary survey, you need to perform a rapid neurologic examination. This includes obtaining a baseline GCS score and pupillary assessment. Check the gross motility of all four extremities to avoid missing and developing hemiplegia. Be on the lookout for deteriorating GCS, developing lateralizing signs, bradycardia, and hypertension.

Management

Effective management of a patient with TBI begins with treating any life-threatening problems identified in the primary survey. Once these problems are addressed, the patient should be rapidly packaged and transported to the nearest facility capable of caring for TBI.

As with any trauma patient, after any exsanguinating hemorrhage has been controlled we need to focus on airway and breathing management. Patients who've experienced a traumatic brain injury may also be dealing with facial injuries. Such injuries can create a difficult airway.

> ## QUICK TIP
>
> As a prehospital care provider, always have backup plans (Plans A, B, and C) to manage the difficult airway. A goal of keeping the TBI patient's SpO$_2$ of at least 90% to 95% is optimal. Because both hypocapnia and hypercapnia can aggravate TBI, controlling the ventilator rate is important.

Hyperventilation of a patient in a controlled fashion may be considered in the specific circumstance of signs of herniation. These signs include:

* Asymmetric pupils
* Dilated and nonreactive pupils
* Extensor posturing or no response on motor examination
* Progressive neurologic deterioration defined as a decrease in the GCS score of more than 2 points in a patient whose initial GCS score was 8 or less.

Mild hyperventilation is defined as an ETCO$_2$ of 30 to 35 mm Hg as measured by capnography or by careful control of the ventilation rate (20 breaths/minute for adults, 25 breaths/minute for children, and 30 breaths/minute for infants less than 1 year of age).

Because hypotension worsens brain ischemia, take standard measures to combat shock. In patients with TBI, the combination of hypoxia and hypotension is associated with a high mortality rate. If shock is present and major internal hemorrhage is suspected, prompt

transport to a trauma center takes priority over other interventions.

Hypovolemic and neurogenic shock should be aggressively treated by resuscitation with intravenous (IV) fluids such as blood products and isotonic crystalloid solutions. To preserve cerebral perfusion, give adequate fluid to maintain a systolic blood pressure of at least 90 mm Hg. For adult TBI patients with normal vital signs and no other suspected injuries, IV fluid at a rate of no more than 125 ml/hour should be administered and adjusted if signs of shock develop. However, don't delay transport to establish IV access.

> ## FOR MORE INFORMATION
>
> Refer to the "Management" section of Chapter 8: Head Trauma.

Refusal of Treatment

You'll often encounter patients who refuse medical treatment and/or transport. These encounters become more complicated when you believe that it's in the patient's best interest to be transported and assessed by a physician. Often, TBI patients with severe mechanisms of injury don't experience the full severity of their injury until hours or days later. Consider patients with an epidural bleed, where there is often a lucid interval, during which the patient feels well, before suffering the potentially fatal effects of hemorrhage hours later.

Patients who've suffered a possible head injury should be evaluated fully with particular attention being paid to their decision-making capacity. Additionally, the following signs and symptoms indicate the need for further medical attention, and this should be communicated to the patient:

* Unequal pupils
* Worsening headache
* Nausea and vomiting
* Drowsiness or difficulty wakening
* Slurring of speech
* Confusion or change in behavior
* Loss of consciousness
* Seizures
* Physical fatigue
* Numbness
* Decreased coordination
* Trouble recognizing people or locations

When you feel that it's in the best interest of the patient to be transported to the hospital for further assessment, and a patient with full decision-making capacity refuses transport, make every attempt to clearly explain the risks of refusal and benefits of care. This includes very direct warnings about the possibility of death and permanent disability that can result from delayed medical care. Contacting medical direction sooner rather than later in these situations can be helpful since some patients are more willing to listen to a physician. If the patient still refuses transport and further treatment, make it clear that he or she can change his or her mind at any time and EMS will be available to return and evaluate them.

When patients don't clearly possess full decision-making capacity, involve medical direction and law enforcement to do what's in the best interest of the patient—transport them to the hospital for further evaluation.

Always follow protocols, medical direction instructions, and local legal statutes when making treatment decisions.

Discuss the Options Early and Often

Discussions regarding the proper course of action to take in scenarios similar to those previously discussed should be had before the incident takes place and should be routinely incorporated into continuing education and initial employee training. The dictum of "first do no harm" should be foundational in the approach to care for all patients encountered by EMS professionals. Patients with questionable capacity are no exception.

Transport

Patients with moderate and severe TBI should be transported directly to a trauma center that can perform CT imaging and provide prompt neurosurgical consultation and intervention (including ICP monitoring, if indicated). If you don't have such a facility in your area, consider aeromedical transport from the scene to an appropriate trauma center.

Take a TBI Lying Down

In general, patients with TBI should be transported in a supine position because of the presence of other injuries. Although elevating the head on the ambulance stretcher or long backboard (reverse Trendelenburg position) may decrease ICP, cerebral perfusion pressure may be jeopardized, especially if the head is elevated higher than 30 degrees.

FOR MORE INFORMATION

Refer to the "Transport" section of Chapter 8: Head Trauma.

PROGRESSIVE CASE STUDY: SUMMARY

While en route to the hospital, you complete the secondary survey with the following findings:

- **X**—Bleeding is controlled.
- **A**—Airway is maintained with a nasal airway and bag-mask device.
- **B**—Breathing is maintained by mildly hyperventilating the patient and keeping the ventilatory rate at 20 breaths/min, watching the capnography, keeping it between 30 to 35 mm Hg. Lungs remain clear.
- **C**—Blood pressure is maintained at 168/90 mm Hg, patient's color improves. Pulse 56 beats/min, strong and regular
- **D**—Serial neurologic exams are done with the patient remaining the same. Patient has decerebrate posturing; GCS 5 (E1, V1, M3).
- **E**—No change

You transport the patient to the closest level I trauma center. A stat CT scan was completed, and the operating room (OR) was mobilized for evacuation of a large epidural hematoma. After surgery, the patient was admitted to the trauma intensive care unit (ICU) with continuing care.

Critical Actions:

- Disability assessment to identify potential life threats
- Determination of the best management for this patient
- Reassessment of interventions

LESSON WRAP-UP

- It is important for EMS practitioners to recognize the signs and symptoms of TBI and make sound decisions on how to treat the patient appropriately.

- EMS treatment of traumatic brain injury is focused on maintaining the patient's oxygenation and perfusion to prevent secondary brain injury.

- It is important to recognize injuries requiring specialized urgent transport to a trauma center.

PROGRESSIVE CASE STUDY RECAP

Part 1

What are the concerning physics of trauma for this patient?	■ The patient fell 3 to 4 ft, and the speed he was traveling could increase the possible injuries. ■ He landed first on his arm and then on his head, and the surface he landed on was unyielding. ■ He also wasn't wearing a helmet or any other safety equipment, which could have prevented or reduced the severity of the fall.
What injuries may the patient have incurred?	■ Skull fractures ■ Facial injuries ■ Other fractures ■ Axial injuries and shear injuries to the cervical spine ■ The arm fracture is concerning, as well, but would be more concerning if it were hemorrhaging. At this point, the arm fracture is a distracting injury in relation to the possible head and spinal injuries.

Part 2

Is there a need for hemorrhage control?	Not with this patient
Is airway management indicated?	With an SpO_2 of 92%, the patient could do with oxygen to bring the oxygen saturation up to 94% or greater. Low flow oxygen at 2 liters/min nasal cannula would be appropriate and titrate to between 94 to 99%.
Is spinal motion restriction indicated?	Yes, until the patient has been evaluated and a decision is made, at a minimum you should complete manual in-line stabilization.
Could this patient have a traumatic brain injury?	Yes.

Part 3

Is airway management necessary for your patient?	The patient's oxygen saturation is 92%, and his $ETCO_2$ is 32 mm Hg. At this point, you should use a nasal cannula vs. nonrebreathing mask, but be prepared to support the patient with a bag-mask device if his condition worsens.

What does the patient's $ETCO_2$ tell you about him?	Changes in pulmonary perfusion, cardiac output, and patient temperature can cause alterations in $ETCO_2$.
How would you manage this patient's initial oxygen needs?	The patient's oxygen saturation is 92%, and 94% and above is optimal. If a nasal cannula isn't sufficient, move to nonrebreathing mask; however, be prepared to bag the patient if his TBI continues to worsen.
Is spinal motion restriction indicated?	Yes. If spinal motion restriction is indicated while managing the airway, be careful that the cervical collar isn't too tight.
Part 4	
What is the appropriate IV access this patient should receive?	You should insert a single IV, reasonable bore (18- or 20-gauge) to optimize chances of success.
What do the unequal pupils indicate in this patient?	Increased intracranial pressure. When ICP increases, it can compress cranial nerve (CN) III which crosses the surface of the tentorium cerebelli. This will cause the nerves' function to be impaired, causing dilation.
What is most likely happening in the brain cavity?	■ TBI ■ Swelling and herniation
What type of injury could be causing the patient to be unconscious?	Axonal injury caused by the patient striking his head and a contra-coup type of injury causing the axons to shear.
Part 5	
How would you prevent secondary brain injury for the patient in this case?	■ Transport the patient at a 30-degree angle. ■ Ensure that the patient does not suffer from hypotension. ■ Ensure that the patient is adequately ventilated and oxygenated. ■ Watch for hypotension, seizures, etc.
What injuries does the patient have that may precipitate secondary brain injury?	■ Oozing dark blood from the right side of the patient's head ■ Confusion ■ Everything that can cause ICP

STUDY QUESTIONS

1. You're called out to an assisted living facility for a 72-year-old woman complaining of a severe headache and experiencing increased confusion. Staff reports she fell out of her wheelchair earlier in the week but didn't appear to be hurt. However, she's become increasingly disoriented over the last day or so. Vital signs show: BP 110/90; heart rate 118 and irregularly regular; ventilation rate 20 and slightly labored; Spo_2 93% on room air. She is taking Coumadin for a clotting issue. Which of the following should you suspect?
   A. Cerebral contusion
   B. Epidural hematoma
   C. Subarachnoid hemorrhage
   D. Subdural hematoma

2. Upon examination, you find the patient responsive to your presence, although she is clearly confused. Motor response shows reduced pain response but normal flexion. What's her GCS score?
   A. 15
   B. 12
   C. 10
   D. 8

3. What does the GCS score indicate?
   A. Mild TBI
   B. Moderate TBI
   C. Severe TBI
   D. No TBI

4. When you examine the patient's pupils, you notice the right one is dilated significantly and her motor response on the left is delayed. What does this suggest?
   A. Coup-countercoup injury
   B. Hyphema
   C. Hypoxia
   D. Uncal herniation

5. Which of the following signs would be most concerning at this point?
   A. A drop in systolic blood pressure to 88 mm Hg
   B. SpO_2 of 93%
   C. A field GCS motor score of 4
   D. Hemiplegia on the left side

6. According to the Monro-Kellie doctrine, what happens to the brain when it is still in a compensated state after a TBI?
   A. CSF, ICP, heart rate, and blood pressure are still within normal range.
   B. CSF increases, ICP decreases, heart rate increases, and blood pressure decreases.
   C. CSF and blood volume decrease, while heart rate and blood pressure are still within normal range.
   D. CSF decreases, ICP increases, heart rate goes down, and blood pressure increases.

ANSWER KEY

Question 1: D
The patient's age, use of a blood thinner, and the fact she fell recently point to a subdural hematoma.

Question 2: B
Eye opening: 4; verbal response: 4; motor response: 4 = 12

Question 3: B
A total GCS score of 13 to 15 likely indicates a mild TBI while a score of 9 to 12 is indicative of moderate TBI. A GCS score of 3 to 8 suggests severe TBI.

Question 4: D
When the medial portion of the temporal lobe (uncus) is pushed toward the tentorium and puts pressure on the brain stem, herniation compresses CN III, the motor tract, and the reticular activating system on the same side, resulting in a dilated or blown pupil on the same side, motor weakness on the opposite side, and respiratory dysfunction, progressing to coma.

Question 5: A
A systolic blood pressure of less than 90 mm Hg indicates secondary brain injury. Her SpO_2 is > 90%, and a motor score of 4 is not as concerning.

Question 6: C
In a compensated state, CSF and blood volume decrease, while heart rate and blood pressure are still within normal range.

REFERENCES AND FURTHER READING

National Association of Emergency Medical Technicians. *PHTLS: Prehospital Trauma Life Support.* 9th ed. Burlington, MA: Public Safety Group; 2019.

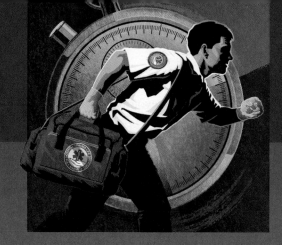

Disability: Spinal Trauma

LESSON OBJECTIVES

- Identify the signs and symptoms of spinal injury and neurogenic shock.
- Describe the pathophysiology of spinal injury and neurogenic shock.
- Demonstrate evidence-based care for spinal injury.
- Identify the indications for spinal motion restriction.
- Select appropriate pain management interventions.

Introduction

Traumatic spine injury (TSI) is potentially life threatening, and its severity depends on where the spine is injured and whether damage includes nearby structures, such as the spinal cord. TSI most often results from high-energy forces but may occur with a lower-energy mechanism of injury (MOI) in vulnerable populations such as older adults.

Causes of TSI include:

- Multi-vehicle collisions: 48%
- Falls: 21%
- Penetrating injuries: 15%
- Sports injuries: 14%
- Other: 2%

QUICK TIP

Injury to the components of the spine may not result in damage to the spinal cord, and, in some cases, the spinal cord, blood vessels, and nerves may be damaged without fracture or dislocation of the vertebrae.

If bony structures and supportive ligaments get damaged, it can lead to instability of the vertebral column, making the spinal cord and other nearby

PROGRESSIVE CASE STUDY: PART 1

You are called to a residential neighborhood on a warm, sunny day in early June for a 24-year-old male who was swimming at a friend's house and dove off the diving board into the pool. Dispatch relays that friends pulled the patient out of the pool when he didn't resurface.

Upon arrival, the scene appears safe—the group of friends gathered around are cooperative, and the decking is a nonslip surface. Bystanders report that the patient dove into the pool and did not come up. Two bystanders pulled the patient from the pool and laid him on the pool deck. You find the patient laying supine at the side of the pool not moving. He states he cannot move his arms or legs and is complaining of neck pain.

Questions:

- What are your concerns about the scene?
- What are your concerns about this patient?
- Do you suspect a traumatic spinal Injury?
- Should manual spinal stabilization be performed?

structures more susceptible to injury unless you restrict spinal motion. Immediate spinal cord damage occurs as a result of the trauma event, or primary injury. Secondary injury can be caused or worsened by motion from an injured spinal column. Failure to suspect, properly assess, and stabilize a patient with a potential spine injury can negatively affect outcome. Prompt recognition and prehospital management of these injuries are important for timely stabilization in the critically injured patient, may guide future diagnostic and management decisions, and will reduce the risk of secondary injury.

A Lifechanging Event

Spinal cord injury (SCI) can have huge effects on physical function, lifestyle, and financial circumstances. When compared to the general population, those who survive the initial SCI generally have a shorter life expectancy.

The spinal cord can be injured at any level, and the two main categories of SCI include complete and incomplete injury.

- Complete SCI affects both sides of the body and results in total loss of all function, including movement and sensation, below the level of the injury. Complete injury at the highest level in the cervical spine is catastrophic and often fatal before emergency personnel arrive on scene.
- Incomplete injury describes any SCI without complete loss of neurologic function. Movement, sensation, or both are preserved but may be asymmetric in a patient with an incomplete SCI. In general, physical dysfunction and long-term impairment increase along the spine, with a cervical spine injury being the most devastating. The loss of motor and sensory function after SCI can range from mild weakness to requiring a wheelchair or even a ventilator.

Understanding the limitations and potential complications of spinal immobilization are important in

---

QUICK TIP

The initial management of a patient with suspected spinal trauma must include aggressive resuscitation and spinal motion restriction to prevent secondary injury and worsened neurologic decline.

---

clinical decision making. The evolution in prehospital management of spine trauma has led to the adoption of evidence-based protocols for spinal motion restriction and management that reduce the complications of immobilization using a rigid backboard, while at the same time limiting spinal motion in patients with an injured spine.

Getting Old Is a Pain in the Back

Osteoporosis, spinal stenosis, and spinal rigidity predispose the geriatric patient to spinal cord injury.

Anatomy & Physiology Review

The spine is a complex structure that:

- Facilitates movement in all three planes
- Disperses the forces from the head and trunk to the pelvis
- Shields the tenuous neurologic tissue of the spinal cord

Vertebral Column

The individual vertebrae of the spine are stacked in an S-shaped column, which allows multidirectional movement while giving maximum support. The spinal column is divided into five individual regions for reference. Beginning at the top and descending downward, these regions are the cervical, thoracic, lumbar, sacral, and coccygeal regions. Each vertebra supports increasing body weight as the vertebrae progress down the spinal column. Appropriately, the vertebrae from C3 to L5 become progressively larger to accommodate the increased weight and workload.

Spinal Cord Anatomy

The spinal cord itself consists of gray matter and white matter. The gray matter consists primarily of the neuronal cell bodies. The white matter contains the long myelinated axons that make up the anatomic spinal tracts and serve as the communication pathways for nerve impulses.

Spinal tracts are divided into two types: ascending and descending.

As the spinal cord continues to descend, pairs of nerves branch off at each vertebra and extend to the various parts of the body.

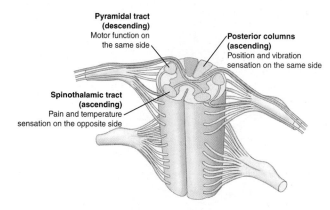

Figure 7B-1 Spinal cord tracts.
© National Association of Emergency Medical Technicians.

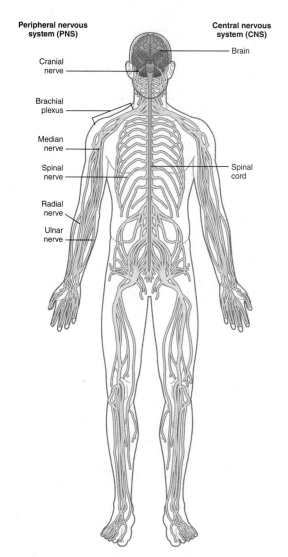

Figure 7B-2 Nerves of the central nervous system (CNS) and peripheral nervous system (PNS).
© National Association of Emergency Medical Technicians.

The spinal cord has 31 pairs of spinal nerves, named according to the level from which they arise. Each nerve has two roots (one dorsal and one ventral) on each side.

- The dorsal root carries information for sensory impulses.
- The ventral root carries motor impulse information.

Stimuli pass between the brain and each part of the body through the spinal cord and respective pairs of these nerves. As they branch from the spinal cord, these nerves pass through a notch in the inferior lateral side of the vertebra, behind the vertebral body, called the intervertebral foramen.

A dermatome is the sensory area on the skin surface innervated by a single dorsal root. Collectively, dermatomes allow the body areas to be mapped out for each spinal level.

Mapping the Landmarks

Dermatomes help determine the level of an SCI. Three landmarks to keep in mind are:

- The clavicles, which are the C4–C5 dermatome
- The nipple level, which is the T4 dermatome
- The umbilicus level, which is the T10 dermatome

Remembering these three levels can help to quickly locate an SCI.

The process of inhalation and exhalation requires chest movement and proper changes in the shape of the diaphragm. The intercostal muscles and accessory respiratory muscles like the trapezius also contribute to breathing. The diaphragm is innervated by the left and right phrenic nerves, which originate from the nerves in the spinal cord between levels C3 and C5. If the spinal cord is injured above the level of C3 or the phrenic nerves are cut, a patient will lose the ability to breathe spontaneously. A patient with this injury may asphyxiate before the arrival of emergency medical services (EMS) unless bystanders initiate rescue breathing.

QUICK TIP

It's critical to maintain control of the airway in a patient with suspected SCI. Positive-pressure ventilation may need to be continued during transport.

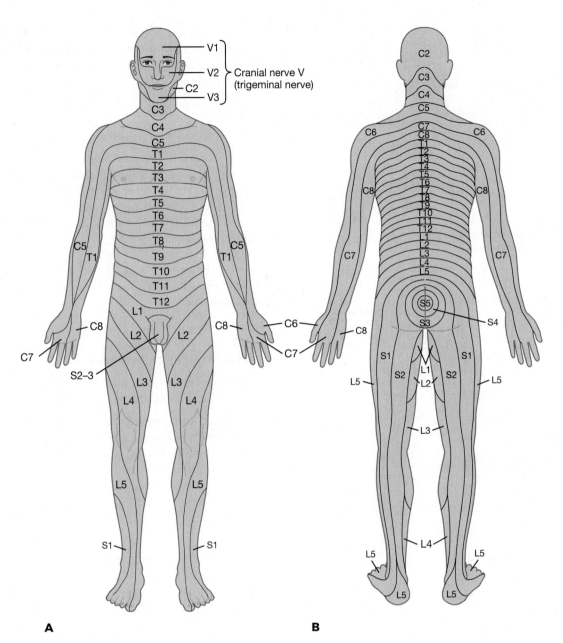

Figure 7B-3 Dermatome map showing the relationship between areas of touch sensation on the skin and the spinal nerves that correspond to these areas. Loss of sensation in a specific area may indicate injury to the corresponding spinal nerve or level of injury of the spinal cord. **A.** Frontal view. **B.** Posterior view.

© National Association of Emergency Medical Technicians.

QUICK TIP

Tongue obstruction, narrowing of airways, and chronic atelectasis create unique challenges for the supine bariatric patient. If full spinal precautions are initiated, ensure frequent airway assessments due to pathophysiologic changes to the structures of the airway and respiratory systems.

FOR MORE INFORMATION

Refer to the "Anatomy and Physiology" section of Chapter 9: Spinal Trauma.

QUICK TIP

Forces acting on the body can stress the osseous and ligamentous structures in the spine beyond their normal limits of motion.

Skeletal Injuries

Various types of injuries can occur to the spine, including:

- Compression fractures, which produce wedge compression or total flattening of the body of the vertebra
- Burst fractures, which can violate the posterior vertebral wall and may produce small fragments of bone that may lie in the spinal canal near the cord
- Subluxation, a partial dislocation of a vertebra from its normal alignment in the spinal column
- Discoligamentous injury, which results from overstretching or tearing of the ligaments and muscles, producing instability between the vertebrae with or without bony injury

While simple compression fractures are usually stable injuries, any of these injuries may result in immediate severe compression or (less commonly) transection of the spinal cord, resulting in irreversible injury. In some patients, however, damage to the vertebrae or ligaments results in an unstable spinal column injury but doesn't produce an immediate SCI. If the fragments in an unstable spine shift position, they may damage the spinal cord secondarily.

Spine Injuries Deficits

A lack of neurologic deficit doesn't rule out a bony fracture or an unstable spine. Although the presence of good motor and sensory responses in the extremities indicates that the spinal cord is currently intact, it does not exclude a damaged vertebra or associated bony, ligamentous, or soft-tissue injury. The majority of patients with spine fractures have no neurologic deficit. A full assessment is required to determine the need for immobilization.

Spinal trauma can be caused from a wide range of mechanisms:

- Axial loading is a result of the spine being compressed, often from the head striking an object or a weighted object striking the head sending the energy into the spine. Compression and axial loading also occur when a patient sustains a fall from a substantial height and lands in a standing position, transferring that energy up the spine.
- Hyperflexion/hyperextension is a result of excessive lateral bending which happens in lateral impacts and posterior impacts causing the spine to move sideways. This movement often results in dislocations and bony fractures.

- Distraction occurs when one part of the spine is stable, and the rest is in longitudinal motion. This pulling apart of the spine can easily cause stretching and tearing of the spinal cord.

QUICK TIP

Distraction-type TSI is a common mechanism in pediatric playground injuries, hangings, and certain types of motor vehicle crashes.

QUICK TIP

Determining the exact mode of failure of the spinal column is difficult since the injury mechanism is often the result of complex force patterns. Always assume that an injury severe enough to produce a fracture or neurologic injury has caused spinal instability until proven otherwise by further clinical and radiographic evaluation.

Spinal Cord Injuries

Primary injury occurs at the time of impact or force application and may cause spinal cord compression, direct SCI (usually from sharp unstable bony fragments or projectiles), and interruption of spinal cord blood flow. Secondary injury occurs after the initial insult and can include swelling, ischemia, or movement of bony fragments.

- **Cord concussion** results from the temporary disruption of spinal cord functions distal to the injury.
- **Cord contusion** involves bruising or bleeding into the tissues of the spinal cord, which may also result in a temporary (and sometimes permanent) loss of spinal cord functions distal to the injury (spinal "shock"). Spinal shock occurs for a variable amount of time after SCI (usually less than 48 hours), resulting in temporary loss of sensory and motor function,

---

QUICK TIP

Cord contusion is often caused by a penetrating type of injury or movement of bony fragments against the spinal cord. The severity of injury is related to the amount of bleeding into the spinal cord tissue. Damage to or disruption of the spinal blood supply can result in local cord tissue ischemia.

muscle flaccidity and paralysis, and loss of reflexes below the level of the SCI.

- **Cord compression** is pressure on the spinal cord caused by swelling of local tissues but also may occur from traumatic disc rupture and bone fragments or development of a compressive hematoma. Cord compression may result in tissue ischemia and in some cases require surgical decompression to prevent a permanent loss of function, so prompt transport for imaging and definitive evaluation is important.
- **Cord laceration** occurs when spinal cord tissue is torn or cut. This type of injury usually results in irreversible neurologic injury.

Spinal cord transection can be categorized as complete or incomplete.

- In complete cord transection, all spinal tracts are interrupted, and all spinal cord functions distal to the site are lost. Because of the additional effects of swelling, determination of the extent of loss of function may not be accurate until 24 hours after the injury. Most complete spinal cord transections result in either paraplegia or quadriplegia, depending on the level of the injury.
- In incomplete cord transection, some tracts and motor/sensory functions remain intact. Prognosis for recovery is greater in these cases than with complete transection.

Intrinsic Causes of Secondary Injury

- Intrinsic causes of secondary injury directly involve CNS tissue and include:
  - Edema: Swelling of the spinal cord compresses nerve fibers, resulting in nerve damage and neurologic deficit.
  - Hematoma: Bleeding within the spinal canal compresses the spinal cord, resulting in nerve damage and neurologic deficit.
  - Increased ICP: The spinal canal is filled with cerebrospinal fluid, thus increased ICP can cause increased pressure within the spinal canal.
  - Seizures: Tonic-clonic movements can worsen spinal cord injuries by movement of displaced vertebrae during the seizure.

Distinctions Aren't Necessary

It's not possible in the prehospital environment to discern whether the resulting neurologic deficit is due to cord contusion, spinal shock, or a more severely damaged spinal cord. Therefore, all suspected SCI patients should be evaluated and managed without consideration of this distinction.

Neurogenic Shock

Spinal shock represents a loss of motor and sensory signal transmission in the spinal cord as a result of injury. Neurogenic shock is a type of distributive shock caused by loss of sympathetic outflow to the heart and peripheral vessels. Without the right amount of sympathetic stimulation, unopposed parasympathetic transmission results in bradycardia and dilation of peripheral arteries and veins. Dilation of arteries results in loss of peripheral systemic vascular resistance, and dilation of veins results in venous pooling. This reduces cardiac preload—the venous return to the right side of the heart. In combination with bradycardia, a serious decrease in cardiac output may occur.

The hypovolemic shock patient presents with tachycardia in response to hypotension, and the skin is cool and clammy as the peripheral blood vessels constrict to shunt blood volume to vital organs in an attempt to maintain blood pressure.

QUICK TIP

Other findings related to the unopposed parasympathetic tone include warm, flushed skin and priapism (abnormal, prolonged erection of the penis) as a result of vasodilation.

Conversely, the classic finding associated with spinal shock is "hypotensive bradycardia" that may require treatment with atropine (or other parasympathetic blocking agent) in addition to other methods of aggressive resuscitation.

Shock: It's Complicated

Patients with SCIs and spinal shock often have other injuries that may result in hypovolemic shock in addition to neurogenic shock, making assessment and management more challenging.

Secondary Injury Resuscitation

Aggressive resuscitation plays a critical role in the prehospital management of SCI-related shock and in reducing neurologic problems and preventing the secondary neurologic damage that stems from loss of autoregulation. Early, aggressive volume and blood pressure augmentation can improve microcirculation and decrease the risk of secondary damage to the cord.

Ideally, initial resuscitation of the SCI patient should include measures to maintain a target MAP of at least 90 mm Hg for 7 days following the injury. This is often accomplished using crystalloids, colloids, or blood products through at least two large-bore intravenous catheters to restore as much neurologic blood flow as possible.

SCI and Hypotension

In the multi-trauma SCI patient, it's important to weigh the potential risk and benefit of permissive hypotension. Given the risks of worsening SCI severity with transient low perfusion states, you should avoid permissive hypotension when SCI is suspected.

You should avoid volume-based resuscitation that includes glucose in the infusion fluids for two reasons:

1. Glucose is metabolized quickly, leaving an excess of free water that is more likely to support the formation of edema.
2. Too much glucose leads to hyperglycemia, which results in increased anaerobic cell metabolism, leading to increased lactate, decreased systemic pH, and a poorer outcome.

It's also important to remember high SCIs (C5 or above) are more likely to require cardiovascular interventions such as vasopressors and pacemakers. Vasomotor sympathetic fibers exit the spinal cord between the first and fourth thoracic vertebrae and may be transected with higher cervical injuries while parasympathetic fibers travel in the vagus nerve outside of the spinal cord to the chest. This results in parasympathetic flow and the paradox of bradycardia with hypotension. While you must be vigilant in your resuscitation efforts for all spinal injuries, it must be overly emphasized in cervical SCI patients to produce the best possible neurologic outcomes for this subset of patients.

QUICK TIP

There is nothing you can do for the initial impact; however, using spinal motion restriction can prevent or reduce additional direct injury from disrupted vertebrae. Secondary injury can worsen the patient's outcome, but you can make a huge difference in patient outcome by recognizing and correcting secondary problems.

Aging and Blunt Trauma

Kyphosis (limiting c-spine range of motion), slower reaction times, polypharmacy, and changes in vision, strength, coordination, and balance predispose the geriatric patient to blunt trauma.

FOR MORE INFORMATION

Refer to the "Pathophysiology" section of Chapter 9: Spinal Trauma.

PROGRESSIVE CASE STUDY: PART 2

Your primary survey reveals the following:

X—No severe external bleeding found
A—Open, patent
B—Fast, normal chest rise
C—Slow, thready radial pulse; skin is pink and warm
D—Glasgow Coma Scale (GCS) = 10 (E4, V5, M6; patient cannot move his arms but can stick out his tongue)
E—Minor abrasion to forehead

Vital signs:

- BP: 82/50 mm Hg
- Heart rate and quality: 54 beats/min, thready radial pulse, weak carotid pulse
- Ventilation rate: 20 breaths/min, diaphragmatic breathing
- SpO_2: 97%/O$_2$
- $ETCO_2$: 42 mm Hg
- Glucose: 100 mg/dl (5.6 mmol/l)
- Skin condition and temperature: warm, pink
- Temperature: 95°F (35°C)

As you do a secondary survey, you note:

- Head: Abrasion to the top of the head with minimal bleeding
- Neck: Pain on palpation to C5 and C6 without deformity/crepitus
- Chest: Lungs clear, diaphragmatic breathing
- Abdomen: Soft, nontender, no signs of trauma
- Pelvis: Stable
- Genitals: Priapism noted
- Back: Unremarkable (assessed when moving patient onto splinting device)
- Extremities: Patient is unable to feel/move his arms or legs.

Questions:

- What pathologic processes explain the patient's presentation?
- What immediate interventions need to be performed?

Assessment

Assess spinal injury in the context of other injuries and conditions present. After ensuring scene safety, the primary survey is the first priority. A rapid scene assessment and history of the event should determine if the possibility of a spinal injury exists, which would require immobilization. You should manually stabilize the patient with a suspected spinal injury in a neutral in-line position until you've assessed the need for continued spinal motion restriction.

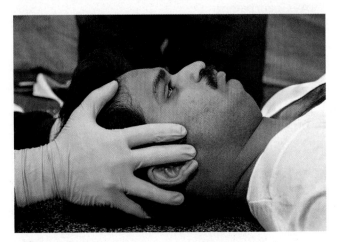

Figure 7B-4 Providing manual cervical spine stabilization.
© National Association of Emergency Medical Technicians.

Maintain the head in that position until the assessment reveals no indication for immobilization, or the manual stabilization is replaced with a spinal motion restriction device, such as cervical collar with a backboard, vacuum mattress, or vest-type device.

If the mechanism of injury is unclear or the scene assessment cannot be adequately performed or is otherwise unreliable, assume the presence of spinal column injury and initiate external immobilization until you can perform a more thorough assessment.

MOI for SCI

The following concepts help clarify the possible effect of energy on the spine when evaluating the potential for injury:

- The head is similar to a bowling ball perched on top of the neck, and its mass often moves in a different direction from the torso, resulting in strong forces being applied to the neck (cervical spine, spinal cord).

- Objects in motion tend to stay in motion, and objects at rest tend to stay at rest (Newton's first law).
- Sudden or violent movement of the upper legs displaces the pelvis, resulting in forceful movement of the lower spine. Because of the weight and inertia of the head and torso, force in an opposite (contra) direction is applied to the upper spine.
- Lack of neurologic deficit does not rule out bone or ligament injury to the spinal column or conditions that have stressed the spinal cord to the limit of its tolerance.

© National Association of Emergency Medical Technicians.

Neurologic Examination

In the field, perform a rapid neurologic examination to identify obvious deficits potentially related to an SCI.

- Ask the patient to move the arms, hands, and legs, and note any inability to do so.
- Check the patient for the presence or absence of sensation, beginning at the shoulders and moving down the body to the feet.

QUICK TIP

You don't need to perform a complete neurologic examination in the prehospital setting, since it won't provide additional information that will affect decisions about prehospital care and serves only to expend precious time on scene and delay transport.

Repeat the rapid neurologic examination after immobilizing the patient, any time the patient is moved, and upon arrival to the receiving facility. This will help identify any changes in patient condition that may have taken place after the primary survey.

Using Mechanism of Injury to Assess SCI

Traditionally, prehospital care providers were taught that suspicion for a spinal injury is based solely on the MOI and that spinal immobilization is required for any patient with a suggestive MOI. Until recently, this generalization caused a lack of clear clinical guidelines for assessment of SCIs. MOI should never be the sole means of determining the need for spinal motion restriction, as it represents only one factor in a multifaceted decision-making process. Assessment of the neck and spine for spinal immobilization should also include assessment of the motor and sensory function, presence of pain or tenderness, and patient reliability as predictors of SCI. In addition, the patient may not complain of pain in the spinal column because of pain associated with a more distracting painful injury, such as a fractured femur.

Don't Get Distracted

The definition of what constitutes a distracting injury remains controversial; however, you should take associated injuries into consideration while assessing a patient for potential TSI and potentially lower the threshold for applying spinal motion restriction if a distracting injury exists.

Alcohol or drugs that the patient may have ingested as well as traumatic brain injury (TBI) may also blunt the patient's perception of pain and mask serious injury. Spinal motion restriction is not indicated in conscious patients with a reliable examination, no neurologic deficit, no neck or back pain, and no significant distracting injury. If any of these factors are positive on examination or are unreliable, continue spinal motion restriction.

Blunt Trauma

As a general guideline, presume the presence of spinal injury and a potentially unstable spine, perform manual stabilization of the cervical spine immediately, and assess the spine to determine the need for immobilization with:

- Any blunt mechanism that produced a violent impact on the head, neck, torso, or pelvis (e.g., assault, entrapment in a structural collapse)
- Incidents that produced sudden acceleration, deceleration, or lateral bending forces to the neck or torso (e.g., moderate- or high-speed motor vehicle crashes, pedestrians struck by vehicle, involvement in explosion)
- Any fall, especially in older adults
- Ejection or fall from any motorized or otherwise powered transportation device (e.g., scooters, skateboards, bicycles, motor vehicles, motorcycles, recreational vehicles)
- Any shallow-water incident (e.g., diving, body surfing)

Other situations often associated with spinal damage include:

- Head injuries with any alteration in level of consciousness
- Significant helmet damage
- Significant blunt injury to the torso
- Impacted or other deceleration fractures of the legs or hips
- Significant localized injuries to the area of the spinal column

These mechanisms of injury should dictate a thorough and complete examination to determine whether spinal motion restriction is indicated. If no indications are found, you can discontinue manual stabilization of the cervical spine.

Penetrating Trauma

Penetrating injury represents a special consideration regarding the potential for spinal trauma. In general, if a patient didn't sustain definite neurologic injury at the moment that the penetrating trauma occurred, there is little concern for subsequent development of an SCI.

Penetrating Injuries

Penetrating injuries by themselves are not indications for spinal immobilization.

Numerous studies have shown that unstable spinal injuries rarely occur from penetrating trauma to the head, neck, or torso, and isolated penetrating injuries by themselves aren't indications for spinal motion restriction. Because of the very low risk of an unstable spinal injury and because the other injuries created by the penetrating trauma often require a higher priority in management, you should not immobilize patients with penetrating trauma.

QUICK TIP

Remember, the failure to suspect, properly assess, and stabilize a patient with a potential spine injury may produce a poor outcome!

Indications for Spinal Motion Restriction

The mechanism of injury can be used as an aid to determine indications for spinal immobilization.

A complete physical assessment coupled with good clinical judgment will guide your decision making.

In 2018, the American College of Surgeons Committee on Trauma, the National Association of EMS Physicians, and the American College of Emergency Physicians updated recommendations regarding the use of spinal motion restriction. Based on these recommendations and current literature, spinal motion restriction should be considered when a blunt mechanism of injury exists with any of the indications listed in the following box.

Indications for Spinal Motion Restriction

- *Midline spinal pain and/or tenderness.* This includes subjective pain or pain on movement, point tenderness, or guarding of the structures in the midline spinal area.
- *Altered level of consciousness or clinical intoxication* (e.g., TBI, under the influence of alcohol or intoxicating substances)
- *Paralysis or focal neurologic signs and/or symptoms* (e.g., numbness and/or motor weakness). This includes bilateral paralysis, partial paralysis, paresis (weakness), numbness, prickling or tingling, and neurogenic spinal shock below the level of the injury. In males, a continuing erection of the penis (priapism) may be an additional indication of SCI.
- *Anatomic deformity of the spine.* This includes any deformity of the spine noted on physical examination of the patient.
- *Presence of a distracting injury*
- *Inability to communicate*

Several important signs and symptoms are concerning for serious spinal trauma. However, the absence of these signs does not definitively rule out spinal injury.

Signs and Symptoms of Spinal Trauma

- Pain in the neck or back
- Pain on movement of the neck or back

- Pain on palpation of the posterior neck or midline of the back
- Deformity of the spinal column
- Guarding or splinting of the muscles of the neck or back
- Paralysis, paresis, numbness, or tingling in the legs or arms at any time after the incident
- Signs and symptoms of neurogenic shock
- Priapism (in male patients)

In an effort to reduce the unnecessary use of spinal motion restriction, particularly with a rigid long backboard, these professional bodies also recommend that immobilization on a backboard is not necessary if the patient meets all of the criteria listed in the following box.

Criteria to Determine When Spinal Motion Restriction Is Unnecessary

- 6.No spine tenderness or anatomic abnormality
- No distracting injury
- No intoxication
- No neurologic findings or complaints

Your main focus is recognizing the indications for spinal motion restriction rather than attempting to clear the spine. Because many patients don't have a spinal injury, use a selective approach when performing spinal motion restriction, especially since spinal immobilization has been shown to produce negative effects in healthy volunteers, including increases in

---

QUICK TIP

The cornerstone to proper spinal care is the same as with all trauma care: superior assessment with appropriate and timely treatment.

FOR MORE INFORMATION

Refer to the "Assessment" section of Chapter 9: Spinal Trauma.

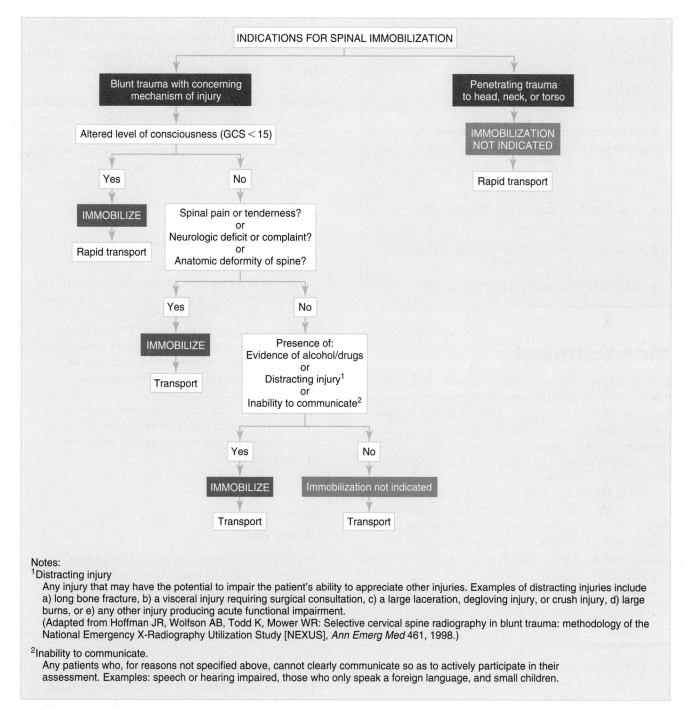

Figure 7B-5 Indications for spinal immobilization.

respiratory effort, skin ischemia, and pain. This selective approach is even more important with the older adult population, who may be more susceptible to skin breakdown and have underlying pulmonary disease. Focus on appropriate indications for performing spinal motion restriction but perform the intervention only if indicated to prevent associated complications. If no indications are present after a careful and thorough examination, there may be no need for spinal immobilization.

Management

If you suspect TSI and spinal motion restriction is appropriate, prepare the patient for transport by safely limiting spinal motion. The goal of spinal immobilization is to limit spinal motion in patients who may have an unstable spinal column injury that could lead to secondary neurologic injury in the context of excess motion.

Fractures of one area of the spine are often associated with fractures of other spinal areas, so the traditional teaching has been that the entire weight-bearing spine (cervical, thoracic, lumbar, and sacral) is considered one entity, and the entire spine is immobilized and supported accordingly.

Patients usually present in one of four general postures:

• Sitting
• Semi-prone
• Supine
• Standing

Taking It Lying Down

The supine position is the most stable position to ensure continued support during handling, carrying, and transporting a patient. It also provides the best access for further examination and additional resuscitation and management of a patient. When the patient is supine, the airway, mouth and nose, eyes, chest, and abdomen can be accessed simultaneously.

If you suspect spinal column injury, you'll need to protect and stabilize the patient's spine immediately and continuously. Techniques and equipment, such as manual stabilization, half-spine boards, immobilization vests, scoop stretchers, proper logroll methods, and rapid extrication with full manual stabilization, are interim techniques used to protect a patient's spine. These techniques allow for a patient's safe movement from the position in which he or she was found until full supine immobilization can be implemented.

Logroll, Scoop, or Backboard?

It's controversial at this point, but some physicians believe that limitation to motion can be done by careful logrolling, using a sheet or sliding board to accomplish transfers, and keeping the patient flat on the ambulance stretcher or cot. Others believe that while such techniques represent the standard of care for protection of the spine within the hospital environment, using a device such as a backboard, scoop litter, or vacuum mattress to reduce the risk of displacement of an unstable spinal segment in the prehospital environment is likely safer.

It's on You

While there's consensus about the general recommendations made here, current scientific research and understanding of spinal motion restriction is incomplete and imperfect. As evidence grows and recommendations continue to evolve, clinical management is ultimately the responsibility of each EMS provider, and you must understand local protocols and discuss the specific techniques to manage these patients with your supervisor and medical director.

There are a number of methods for performing spinal motion restriction.

The Backboard Debate

While backboards provide motion restriction of the entire spine, it's important to understand a number of facts about the backboard itself. Being placed onto a rigid board is an extremely uncomfortable experience. In addition, being immobilized on a rigid backboard leads to a significant amount of pressure being placed on areas in contact with the board. Over time, circulation to these areas becomes compromised, leading to skin ischemia, necrosis, and decubitus ulcers. You should place padding under the patient and to minimize the amount of time a patient spends on the board. In addition, some patients, especially those who are obese, may experience respiratory compromise from being strapped supine onto a board.

These concerns have led to a growing move to decrease or completely end the use of the backboard or to remove patients from the board once the patient has been placed on the stretcher. While it's clear that too many patients are unnecessarily immobilized based solely on the MOI, like any intervention, you must carefully consider all your management strategies.

It's certainly possible to maintain spinal alignment and limit motion by simply laying a patient on an ambulance cot in a supine position with a cervical collar in place. This is the technique used to immobilize patients in the hospital even after an unstable cervical or thoracolumbar injury has been formally diagnosed.

Alignment Without Immobilization

Given that most EMS transport times in the United States are short and that the length of time patients in the hospital need to maintain spinal motion restriction or immobilization is long, the degree of discomfort associated with use of a backboard in the hospital is much greater than in the prehospital environment, and the risk of secondary spinal column displacement and secondary neurologic injury is small. This is the reason that patients should be (and routinely are) removed from backboards or immobilization devices soon after arrival at hospitals or trauma centers.

Eliminating the use of long backboards in the prehospital setting is occurring more frequently in the United States and Europe with no evidence of an increase in the incidence of catastrophic secondary neurologic injury.

You can use a scoop stretcher or vacuum mattress as an alternative to a rigid long backboard, since they're often easier to apply and may be more comfortable. You need to immobilize the head, neck, torso, and pelvis in a neutral in-line position to prevent any further movement of an unstable spine.

QUICK TIP

While some EMS agencies in the United States are beginning to consider elimination of the use of long backboards, others have chosen to modify their use of backboarding techniques to limit discomfort rather than expose patients to the potential risk of secondary catastrophic injury. Be aware of the changes in your system, and remain up to date on the latest evidence and protocol changes.

QUICK TIP

Spinal immobilization follows the common principle of fracture management: immobilizing the joint above and the joint below an injury. Because of the anatomy of the spine, this principle of immobilization must be extended beyond just the joint above and below a suspected vertebral injury. The joint above the spine means the head and the joint below means the pelvis.

The Scoop on the Scoop

The scoop stretcher has traditionally been made out of metal (aluminum or other lightweight metals), but modern plastics are now more commonly used. It's a two-part device, allowing the separated halves to be placed under each side of the patient without the need for much manipulation. After fastening the two halves together, the patient can be lifted and transferred to an ambulance stretcher or vacuum mattress.

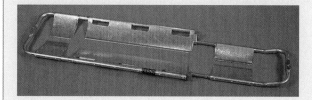

Figure 7B-6 Scoop stretcher.
© Jones and Bartlett Learning. Courtesy of MIEMSS.

The Vacuum Mattress Splint

The vacuum mattress is a transport and immobilization tool used after the patient has been transferred to it with a scoop stretcher. The splint is an airtight polymer bag filled with small polystyrene balls and a valve. When the air inside the vacuum mattress is sucked out, the atmospheric pressure outside presses the balls together, forming a rigid "bed" for the patient that molds to the patient's body contours.

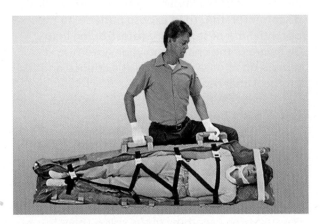

Figure 7B-7 Vacuum mattress splint.
Courtesy of Hartwell Medical.

The vacuum mattress is more comfortable compared to the long rigid backboard and, similar to most backboards, is x-ray penetrable, so the patient doesn't need to be removed while being evaluated in the emergency department.

> ### The Arm Bone's Connected to the Shoulder Girdle
>
> Moderate anterior flexion or extension of the arms can cause significant movement of the shoulder girdle. Any movement or angulation of the pelvis results in movement of the sacrum and of the vertebrae attached to it. For example, lateral movement of both legs together can result in angulation of the pelvis and lateral bending of the spine.

In some instances, the patient may benefit from spinal precautions rather than complete spinal motion restriction. Spinal precautions can be performed by applying a rigid cervical collar and firmly securing the patient to the stretcher. This is likely more appropriate in:

- Patients who are ambulatory on the scene
- Patients who have mild to moderate neck pain, are reliable, have no neurologic deficit or complaints, and who have no back or other thoracolumbar pain

- Patients for whom a backboard or other spinal restricting device is not otherwise indicated based on presence of distracting injury, decreased level of consciousness, or evidence of intoxication

> ### Be Flexible With Immobilization
>
> Often, we place too much focus on particular immobilization devices without an understanding of the principles of immobilization and how to modify these principles to meet individual patient needs. Specific devices and immobilization methods can be safely used only with an understanding of the anatomic principles that apply to all methods and equipment. Any inflexible, detailed method for using a device will not meet the varying conditions found in the field.

General Method

Regardless of the specific equipment or method used, the management of any patient with an unstable spine should follow these principles:

1. Move the patient's head into a proper neutral in-line position (unless contraindicated; see next section). Continue manual support and in-line stabilization without interruption.
2. Evaluate the patient by performing the primary survey and provide any immediately required intervention.
3. Check the patient's motor ability, sensory response, and circulation in all four extremities, if the patient's condition allows.
4. Examine the patient's neck, and measure and apply a properly fitting, effective cervical collar.
5. Depending on the situation and how critical the patient's injuries are, either position a short backboard or vest-type device on the patient or use a rapid extrication maneuver if the patient is in a motor vehicle. Place the patient on a long backboard or other appropriate immobilization device if he or she is lying on the ground.
6. Immobilize the patient's torso to the device so that it cannot move up, down, left, or right.
7. Evaluate and pad behind the adult patient's head or pediatric patient's chest as needed.
8. Immobilize the patient's head to the device, maintaining a neutral in-line position.
9. Once the patient is on the immobilization device (if a short device is used), immobilize the legs so that they cannot move anteriorly or laterally.
10. Secure the patient's arms if indicated.

11. Reevaluate the primary survey, and reassess the patient's motor ability, sensory response, and circulation in all four extremities, if the patient's condition allows.

Manual In-Line Stabilization of the Head

Once you've determined from the MOI that an injured spine may exist, the first step is to provide manual in-line stabilization. Grasp the patient's head, and carefully move it into a neutral in-line position unless contraindicated. A proper neutral in-line position is maintained without any significant traction on the head and neck. Maintain the head in the manually stabilized, neutral in-line position until you can complete mechanical immobilization of the torso and head or the examination reveals no need for spinal immobilization.

Contraindications

If careful movement of the head and neck into a neutral in-line position results in any of the following, stop the movement immediately:

- Resistance to movement
- Neck muscle spasm
- Increased pain
- Commencement or increase of a neurologic deficit, such as numbness, tingling, or loss of motor ability
- Compromise of the airway or ventilation

QUICK TIP

Don't attempt neutral in-line movement if a patient's injuries are so severe that the head presents with such misalignment that it no longer appears to extend from the midline of the shoulders. In these situations, the patient's head must be immobilized in the position in which it was initially found. Fortunately, such cases are rare.

QUICK TIP

You must practice your immobilization skills in hands-on sessions using mock patients before use with real patients. At least one study has shown that appropriate immobilization was not performed in a significant number of patients with potential spinal injury.

When practicing or evaluating new methods or equipment, consider the following criteria for measuring how effective the intervention has been at restricting spinal motion:

1. Initiate manual in-line stabilization immediately, and maintain it until it is replaced mechanically.
2. Check neurologic function distally.
3. Apply an effective, properly sized cervical collar.
4. Secure the torso before the head.
5. Prevent movement of the torso up or down the device.
6. Prevent movement of the upper and lower torso left or right on the immobilization device.
7. Ensure ties crossing the chest do not inhibit chest excursion or result in ventilatory compromise.
8. Effectively immobilize the head so that it cannot move in any direction.
9. Provide padding behind the head, if necessary.
10. Maintain the head in a neutral in-line position.
11. Ensure that nothing inhibits or prevents the mouth from being opened and that sufficient access to the airway is present to effectively allow the provider to maintain and protect airway integrity.
12. Immobilize the legs so that they cannot move anteriorly, rotate, or move from side to side, even if the board and patient are rotated to the side.
13. Maintain the pelvis and legs in a neutral in-line position.
14. Ensure that the arms are appropriately secured to the device or torso.
15. Ensure that any ties or straps do not compromise distal circulation in any limb.
16. Reevaluate the patient if bumped, jostled, or in any way moved in a manner that could compromise an unstable spine while the device was being applied.
17. Complete the procedure within an appropriate time frame.
18. Recheck distal neurologic function.

The selection of a specific method and specific equipment should be based on the situation, the patient's condition, and available resources.

Don't Do That

The most common immobilization errors include:

1. Failing to adequately provide spinal motion restriction such that the torso can move significantly up or down on the board device or the head can still move excessively.

2. Improperly sizing or improperly applying the cervical collar.
3. Immobilizing the patient with the head hyperextended. The most common cause is a lack of appropriate padding behind the head.
4. Immobilizing the head before the torso or readjusting the torso straps after the head has been secured. This causes movement of the device relative to the torso, which results in movement of the head and cervical spine.
5. Inadequately padding. Failure to fill the voids under a patient can allow for inadvertent movement of the spine, resulting in additional injury as well as increased discomfort for the patient.
6. Placing someone in spinal immobilization who does not meet immobilization criteria.
7. Taking excessive time to achieve immobilization in the context of a physiologically unstable or potentially unstable patient.
8. Using overly aggressive immobilization techniques that fail to prioritize maintaining and protecting airway integrity.

Complete spinal motion restriction is an uncomfortable experience for the patient. Spinal immobilization is a balance between the need to protect and immobilize the spine completely, the need to maintain and protect airway access, the need to expeditiously initiate transport, and the need to make it tolerable for the patient. That's why proper evaluation is indicated.

QUICK TIP

In the event the pediatric patient shows signs and symptoms of spinal cord injury, despite a negative CT or x-ray, maintain full spinal precautions. SCIWORA (Spinal Cord Injury Without Radiographic Abnormality) can occur due to the immature structure of the pediatric spinal cord. An MRI may be needed in order to fully clear the pediatric patient.

Rapid Extrication Versus Short Device for the Seated Patient

You'll need to base the decision to use a rapid extrication technique over a short device on the clinical presentation of the patient, the findings during the primary survey, and the situation at the scene. If the patient has

critical injuries; has airway, breathing, or circulation issues; or is in shock or impending shock, rapid extrication techniques and rapid transport are appropriate. The benefit in rapidly accessing the patient and treating these conditions outweighs the risk of the extrication procedure. Fortunately, few patients fall into this category. In most stable patients, a short device can be used.

Special Considerations

When using backboards on bariatric trauma patients, you need to ensure not to exceed safe operating limits. Also, additional personnel must be present to help lift and extricate bariatric patients to avoid causing further injury to the patient or prehospital care providers.

FOR MORE INFORMATION

Refer to the "Management" section of Chapter 9: Spinal Trauma.

PROGRESSIVE CASE STUDY: PART 4

Upon further reassessment, you find the following:

- BP: 92/54 mm Hg
- Heart rate and quality: 54 beats/min, thready radial pulse
- Ventilation rate: 20 breaths/min, diaphragmatic breathing
- SpO_2: 97%/O_2
- $ETCO_2$: 42 mm Hg
- Glucose: 100 mg/dl (5.6 mmol/l)
- Skin condition and temperature: pink, warm
- Temperature: 95°F (35°C)
- Pain: 4/10

Questions:

- Could this patient have been given pain medications?
- Could atropine have been used for the bradycardia?
- Should steroids be used as a treatment for spinal cord injuries?
- Is there a risk for respiratory compromise?

Prolonged Transport

As with other injuries, the prolonged transport of patients with suspected or confirmed spine and spinal cord injuries presents special issues. While backboards may be valuable for transfers over short distances or duration, they should not be used as immobilization devices for longer than 30 minutes. Such efforts should help reduce the risk for the development of pressure ulcers in a patient with SCI.

QUICK TIP

For transports that will exceed 30 minutes, consider using a scoop stretcher to carefully lift a patient, removing the long backboard, and then placing the patient down onto the ambulance cot.

You should pad any areas where there might be pressure on the patient's body, especially over bony prominences. Patients who are immobilized in a supine position are at risk for aspiration if they vomit. In the event the patient begins to vomit, immediately tip the backboard and patient onto the side. Keep suction near the patient's head so it's readily accessible if vomiting occurs. Insertion of a gastric tube (either nasogastric or orogastric), if allowed, and the judicious use of antiemetic medications may help reduce this risk.

Patients with high SCIs may have involvement of their diaphragm and accessory respiratory muscles, predisposing them to respiratory failure. Impending respiratory failure may be aggravated and hastened by straps placed across the trunk for spinal immobilization that further restrict respiration. Prior to initiating a prolonged transport, double-check that the patient's torso is secured at the shoulder girdle and at the pelvis and that any straps don't limit chest wall excursion.

When the Signs Are Low

Patients with high SCIs may experience hypotension from loss of sympathetic tone (neurogenic "shock"). Although these patients rarely suffer from widespread hypoperfusion, crystalloid boluses are usually sufficient to restore blood pressure to normal.

Another hallmark of a high cervical spine injury is bradycardia. If associated with significant hypotension, bradycardia may be treated with intermittent doses of atropine, 0.5 to 1.0 mg, administered intravenously.

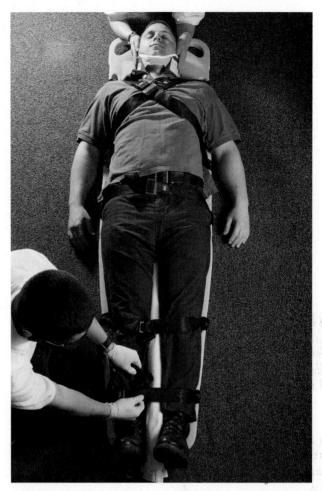

Figure 7B-8 Caudad movement of the torso can be prohibited by use of straps that pass snugly around the pelvis and legs.
© Jones & Bartlett Learning. Photographed by Darren Stahlman.

Patients with spinal injuries may have significant back pain or pain from associated fractures. You can manage pain with small doses of intravenous narcotics titrated until pain is relieved. Narcotics may exaggerate the hypotension associated with neurogenic shock.

Patients with SCIs lose some ability to regulate body temperature, and this effect is more pronounced with injuries higher in the spinal cord. Keep in mind that these patients are sensitive to the development of hypothermia, especially when they're in a cold environment. Keep patients warm (normothermic), but remember that covering them with too many blankets may lead to hyperthermia.

Placing Pregnant Patients

Occasionally a pregnant patient will require spinal immobilization. Depending on the gestational age, placing the patient in a fully supine position may cause compression of the inferior vena cava by the gravid uterus, leading to a decrease in venous blood return to the heart, and decreasing the mother's blood pressure. Once secured, tip the backboard on an angle to place the patient in a relative left lateral position (left side down with blanket or padding under the right side of the patient sufficient enough to support this position).

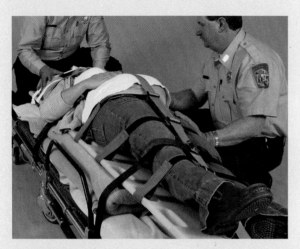

Figure 7B-9 Tipping a pregnant female onto her left side helps displace the uterus from the inferior vena cava and improves blood return to the heart, thus restoring blood pressure.

© Jones and Bartlett Learning. Courtesy of MIEMSS.

FOR MORE INFORMATION

Refer to the "Prolonged Transport" section of Chapter 9: Spinal Trauma.

PROGRESSIVE CASE STUDY: SUMMARY

The patient was transported by ground ambulance to a level I trauma center where he was stabilized. He underwent surgical intervention for a cervical spine fracture at C5 and C6, with no irreversible cord damage.

The patient was discharged several weeks later to a rehabilitation facility and discharged home 3 months later with almost full mobility; however, he will require further rehabilitation over time.

Critical Actions:

- Disability assessment to identify potential life threats
- Determination of the best management for this patient
- Reassessment of interventions

LESSON WRAP-UP

- Spinal motion restriction should be determined by MOI and through a thorough patient examination.
- Immobilization should focus on appropriate treatment and reducing secondary injury to the spine.
- Neurogenic shock should be treated as appropriate to maintain good perfusion to the spinal cord to prevent further damage and a poor neurologic outcome.

PROGRESSIVE CASE STUDY RECAP

Part 1	
What are your concerns about the scene?	The incident may involve a possible near drowning, traumatic brain injury, and spinal injuries.
	Scene safety issues include:
	■ Possibly intoxicated friends
	■ High emotion
	■ Panicky friends
	■ Slippery surfaces
	The MOI may involve the patient striking his head on the diving board or the side of the pool.

What are your concerns about this patient?	Because the patient was pulled from the pool, airway and breathing should be concerns. Also, since the patient is lying exposed and wet, hypothermia can be a concern.
Do you suspect a traumatic spinal Injury?	Yes. ■ There's an abrasion on his forehead suggesting significant force into the pool wall/bottom ■ There is no movement of the patient's limbs ■ He has neck pain and no mobility at his limbs ■ His skin is pink and warm with a thready pulse suggesting compensated vasodilation—loss of nervous control of the blood vessels.
Should manual spinal stabilization be performed?	Yes, you should perform manual in-line stabilization because of the MOI and because the patient can't move his extremities.

Part 2

What pathologic processes explain the patient's presentation?	The patient has a spinal injury at the level of C5 and C6, based on assessment findings.
What immediate interventions need to be performed?	Consider spinal motion restriction since the patient has a neurologic deficit and a suspected spinal injury.

Part 3

Is the patient reliable to evaluate his condition?	Altered mental status can affect a patient's ability to provide reliable information about his or her condition. In this case, the patient is oriented and mentating appropriately, so he is reliable to evaluate his condition.
What conditions would be concerning and make you doubt a patient's reliability?	Altered mental status, districting painful injuries, and communication barriers are all things you need to consider. ■ Patients who have sustained a TBI and have altered mental status cannot be adequately evaluated and should be immobilized. ■ Manage patients under the influence of drugs or alcohol as if they had a spinal injury until they're calm, cooperative, and sober and physical exam is normal. A reliable patient is calm and cooperative and has a completely normal mental status.
How should this patient be packaged for transport?	Use a spinal motion restriction device that minimizes further secondary injury to the patient. Use a backboard, scoop, or vacuum splint to lift the patient to the stretcher—remove the backboard or scoop once the patient is on the stretcher.
How would packaging be different if the patient were unconscious?	If the patient were unconscious, he would need to remain fully restrained on a backboard or scoop stretcher to prevent movement.

(continued)

PROGRESSIVE CASE STUDY RECAP (*CONTINUED*)

What condition could be causing the patient's vital signs to be abnormal?	The patient could be experiencing spinal shock.
How should this patient be managed?	Consider spinal motion restriction along with an IV to maintain a systolic BP of at least 90 mm Hg. In the event of spinal shock, the patient may require a parasympathetic blocking agent (such as atropine) in addition to IV fluids to manage hypotensive bradycardia.
Part 4	
Could this patient have been given pain medications?	Many common anesthetic agents, including morphine and other opioids, can reduce cardiac output due to negative inotropic effects on cardiac muscle. While pain control in a trauma patient is important, these agents must be used judiciously to allow for adequate cord perfusion and oxygenation. Patients with high spinal cord injuries are more sensitive to the effects of sedatives and analgesics.
Could atropine have been used for the bradycardia?	Patients with high spinal cord injuries may experience hypotension from loss of sympathetic tone (neurogenic shock). Although these patients rarely suffer from widespread hypoperfusion of their tissues, crystalloid solution boluses are generally sufficient to restore their blood pressure to normal. Vasopressors are rarely, if ever, necessary to treat neurogenic shock. Another hallmark of a high cervical spine injury is bradycardia. If associated with significant hypotension, bradycardia may be treated with intermittent doses of atropine, 0.5 to 1.0 microgram (mcg), administered intravenously.
Should steroids be used as a treatment for spinal cord injuries?	Steroids are not currently recommended in the prehospital management of spinal cord injury. Several older studies suggested that high doses of the steroid methylprednisolone improve the neurologic outcome of some patients when started within 8 hours of the injury. Spinal cord injuries in children or those resulting from penetrating trauma were not studied, and steroids are never indicated for neurologic deficits resulting from stab or gunshot wounds. The complications associated with steroid administration may significantly outweigh any benefit.

STUDY QUESTIONS

1. You are responding to a call for 25-year-old, fit and healthy female who fell off a mountain bike. Upon arrival, you find the patient walking around. She is alert but complaining of pain in her clavicle and on her right side when she inhales. You notice that her helmet is split in two. What's the first thing you need to do?
    A. Complete a review of the ABCs
    B. Check motor and sensory function
    C. Perform manual in-line stabilization
    D. Place her on a backboard

2. During primary survey, you find the following:
   - LOC: alert and oriented. Speaking in full sentences
   - GCS: 15
   - Airway: good air entry to bases
   - Breathing: bilateral
   - Circulation: skin warm, pink, dry
   - Pulse rate: 112 strong and regular
   - BP: 90/42
   - Pain: Patient complains of severe pain at clavicle site and pain on inspiration at site of possible fractured ribs. No other injuries detected

   What's your next step?
   A. Apply a cervical collar and in-line immobilization device
   B. Treat for hypovolemic shock
   C. Apply an arm sling for the clavicle injury
   D. Administer pain medication

3. Which body part should you secure first?
   A. Head
   B. Torso
   C. Legs
   D. Pelvis

4. How should you immobilize the patient's torso?
   A. Strap the upper torso with two straps in an X shape where a strap goes from each side of the board over the shoulder, then across the upper chest and through the opposite armpit, to fasten to the board on the armpit side.
   B. Fasten one strap to the board and pass it through one armpit, then across the upper chest and through the opposite armpit, to fasten to the second side of the board.
   C. Place backpack-type loops around each shoulder through the armpit and fasten the ends of each loop in the same handhold.
   D. Secure three straps snugly over the lower third of the thorax.

5. What type of padding should you provide for this patient as you immobilize her?
   A. Use compressible padding under the shoulders and torso to prevent hyperflexion.
   B. Use firm padding between the back of the head and the backboard to prevent hyperextension.
   C. Do not use any padding. It can cause extension or flexion in the neck.
   D. No padding but to avoid decreased venous return, you should tip the backboard to a left lateral position.

6. While attempting to lay the patient supine for spinal immobilization she becomes increasingly distressed and complains of shortness of breath and difficulty breathing. The fractured clavicle appears to move distally and increases the difficulty of breathing as the patient lays back. What should you do?
   A. Tip the backboard to a left lateral position.
   B. Raise the back of the stretcher.
   C. Let her sit up in a position of comfort.
   D. Administer morphine.

ANSWER KEY

Question 1: C
Because there's a possibility of spinal injury, you should bring the patient's head into a neutral in-line position.

Question 2: A
Although the patient's GCS is normal, she does have a distracting injury and the state of her helmet indicates possible spinal compression/flexion, so you should immobilize the patient.

Question 3: B
When immobilizing a patient, you should secure the torso first, then the head, the legs, and the pelvis.

Question 4: C
Because the patient has a clavicle injury, you should place backpack-type loops around each shoulder through the armpit and fasten the ends of each loop in the same handhold. The straps remain near the lateral edges of the upper torso and do not cross the clavicles.

Question 5: B
Because the patient is an adult, you should use firm padding between the back of the head and the backboard to prevent hyperextension. You would pad a child's shoulder and torso to prevent hyperflexion, and you would tip the backboard for a pregnant patient to prevent decrease venous return.

Question 6: B
Since laying the patient increases the risk of airway/ventilation problems, sitting her up slightly fundamentally maintains spinal alignment while reducing the ventilation issues.

REFERENCES AND FURTHER READING

National Association of Emergency Medical Technicians. *PHTLS: Prehospital Trauma Life Support*. 9th ed. Burlington, MA: Public Safety Group; 2019.

Sechrest, R. Cervical Spinal Anatomy. https://www.youtube.com/watch?v=RNUpMNd_u1U. Accessed November 13, 2018.

SKILL STATIONS

Rapid Extrication With Three or More Providers

1. Once the decision is made to extricate a patient rapidly, manual in-line stabilization of the patient's head and neck in a neutral position is initiated by your partner. This is best accomplished from behind the patient. If your partner is unable to get behind the patient, manual in-line stabilization can be accomplished from the side. Whether from behind the patient or the side, the patient's head and neck are brought into a neutral alignment, a rapid assessment of the patient is performed, and a properly sized cervical collar is applied.

2. While manual in-line stabilization is maintained, you control the patient's upper torso and lower torso and legs. Rotate the patient in a series of short, controlled movements.

3. Continue to rotate the patient in short, controlled movements until control of manual in-line stabilization can no longer be maintained from behind and inside the vehicle.

4. A second partner assumes manual in-line stabilization from the first partner while standing outside of the vehicle.

5. The first partner can now move outside the vehicle and reassume manual in-line stabilization from the second partner.

6. The rotation of the patient is continued until the patient can be lowered out of the vehicle door opening and onto a spinal motion restriction device.

7. If the scene is unsafe, the patient should be moved to a safe area before being secured to the spinal motion restriction device.

Two-Provider Rapid Extrication

1. Your partner approaches the car and maintains manual in-line stabilization from the driver's side through an open window, if possible.

2. Enter the car from the passenger side and take over manual in-line stabilization from the front. Your partner places an appropriately sized cervical collar on the patient.

3. Your partner prepares and positions the needed equipment:
   - Long-rolled blanket or similar device
   - Ambulance stretcher
   - Spinal motion restriction device

4. Your partner positions the stretcher so the height matches the seat in the car.

5. Your partner wraps the rolled blanket around the cervical collar and under the patient's arms.

6. Your partner grasps the ends of the blanket roll and begins to pivot the patient.

7. You now can release the manual in-line stabilization and guide the patient's legs toward the passenger side of the vehicle.

8. You and your partner continue to pivot the patient until they are in alignment with the spinal motion restriction device, and then longitudinally slide the patient into position and secure on spinal motion restriction device.

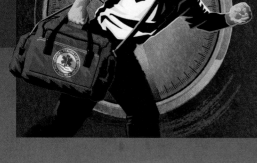

Special Considerations

LESSON OBJECTIVES
· Discuss burn assessment and treatment.
· Learn to assess and treat pediatric trauma patients.
· Apply adult trauma treatment concepts to pediatric trauma patients.
· Apply adult trauma treatment concepts to geriatric trauma patients.
· Choose the most appropriate pain management intervention based on clinical findings.

Introduction

Every patient is not the same—especially when it comes to pediatric and geriatric patients. As with all aspects of special population care, proper assessment and management require a thorough understanding of not only the unique characteristics of age group development but also unique mechanisms of injury.

Children: Little Adults?

The adage holds true that "children are not just little adults." Children have distinct, reproducible patterns of injury, different physiologic responses, and special treatment needs based on their physical and psychosocial development at the time of injury.

With an ever-growing population of older adults, an increasing number of geriatric patients are suffering traumatic injuries. Trauma is the fourth leading cause of death in people between age 55 and 64 and is the ninth leading cause of death in those aged 65 years and older. Specific mechanisms and patterns of injury are also unique to the older adult population. Although motor vehicle crashes are the overall leading cause of trauma deaths, falls are the main mechanism of death in patients older than 75 years.

This lesson dives into some of the major differences in our younger and older patients along with the specialty care that is needed for burn victims and obstetric trauma patients.

QUICK TIP

Although the unique characteristics of specialty care are important for you to understand, the basic life support (BLS) and advanced life support (ALS) treatment approach using the primary and secondary surveys is the same for every patient, regardless of age or size.

PROGRESSIVE CASE STUDY 1: PART 1

Your unit is dispatched for a 2-year-old male with a burn injury to the hand. The patient's caregiver is a babysitter who reports the child was crawling on the counter and placed his hand in a pot of water that was boiling on the stove. Law enforcement is on the scene speaking with the caregiver, who is holding the patient. The child is squirming and attempting to get away from the caregiver. He has a visible burn to the entire left hand ending at the level above the wrist as well as redness and blisters to his face. There is an audible stridor as you enter the room. The child appears pale, and his skin is cool and dry to the touch.

Your primary survey reveals the following:

- **X**—No exsanguinating hemorrhage noted
- **A**—Audible stridor present
- **B**—Ventilation rate of 32 breaths/min; clear breath sounds bilaterally
- **C**—Rapid pulse rate present; skin cool, pale, and dry
- **D**—Pediatric Glasgow Coma Scale (GCS) score of 15 (E4, V5, M6)
- **E**—Burn to the left hand, red in color, wet in appearance, and ending at the level of the wrist. The caregiver has an ice pack applied to the burned hand. The child is shivering.

Questions:

- How common are burns in pediatric patients?
- Which types of burns are the most common?
- What would lead you to suspect this was an intentionally caused burn injury?
- What population of patients is at increased risk for burn injuries?
- How do we estimate burn depth?
- What are the unique anatomic and physiologic characteristics of this patient that are of concern?

Burns

Scald burns from hot liquids are the most common burns to children and older adults. Older adults and children are the most susceptible populations to burn injury.

Pathophysiology of Burn Injury

When skin gets burned, it immediately breaks down, affecting temperature regulation, protection against infection, and maintenance of fluid homeostasis. A burn injury interferes with systemic circulation because of the loss of vascular wall integrity and the resultant loss of protein into the interstitium. More fluid moves into the interstitial space because of increased capillary permeability. This causes rapid fluid shifts from the intravascular compartment.

Burns Are Traumatic

With large burn injuries, the dramatic loss of fluids, electrolytes, and protein results in loss of effective circulating plasma volume, massive edema formation, decreased end-organ perfusion, and depressed cardiovascular function.

The consensus is to give the least amount of fluid necessary to maintain adequate end-organ perfusion, and the replacement of extracellular salt lost in the burned tissue is essential.

QUICK TIP

Several different resuscitation formulas are available, with the biggest difference being the composition of resuscitation fluid.

FOR MORE INFORMATION

Refer to the "Pathophysiology of Burn Injury" section of Chapter 13: Burn Injuries.

Burn Characteristics

A burn injury is caused by heat damaging the skin, subcutaneous tissue, fat, muscle, and even bone. Acute thermal injury causes tissue necrosis (tissue death) at the center of injury with progressively less damage at the outer edges. The depth of the injury depends on the degree of heat exposure and depth of heat penetration.

Injury to the skin occurs in two phases:

- Immediate injury is from acute thermal exposure, resulting in immediate loss of plasma membrane integrity and protein denaturation.

- Delayed injury results from inadequate resuscitation, desiccation, edema, and wound infection.

> ### Timing Is Everything
>
> Timely and appropriate burn care, including systemic fluid resuscitation and avoiding vasoconstriction is critical in prevention of necrosis in this zone of injury. Failure to resuscitate the patient appropriately results in death of the cells in the injured tissue leading to tissue necrosis.

> ### QUICK TIP
>
> A common mistake that damages the zone of stasis is the application of ice by a bystander or prehospital care provider. Ice applied to the skin in an effort to stop the burning process can cause vasoconstriction, preventing reestablishment of blood flow that is critically needed for the injured tissue.

Burn Depth

Estimating burn depth can be deceptively hard for even the most experienced prehospital care provider. Often, the surface of a burn may appear to be partial thickness at first glance, but later, after debridement in the hospital, the superficial epidermis separates, revealing a white, full-thickness burn eschar underneath.

> ### QUICK TIP
>
> Often, it is best to simply tell patients that the injury is either superficial or deep and that further evaluation is required to determine ultimate burn depth.

Superficial Burns

Superficial burns involve only the epidermis and are characterized as red and painful. These burns extend into the papillary dermis and characteristically form blisters. These wounds blanch with pressure, and blood flow to this area is increased compared to adjacent normal skin. Burns of this depth are not included when calculating the percentage of total body surface area (TBSA) that is burned or used for fluid administration.

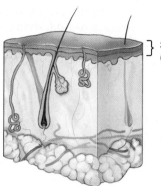

Figure 8-1 Superficial burn.
© National Association of Emergency Medical Technicians.

Partial-Thickness Burns

Partial-thickness burns, once referred to as second-degree burns, involve the epidermis and portions of the underlying dermis. They can be further classified as either superficial or deep.

Partial-thickness burns will appear as blisters or as denuded burned areas with a glistening or wet-appearing base.

> ### Blisters
>
> Much discussion has been generated about blisters, including whether or not to open and debride them and how to approach the blister associated with partial-thickness burns.
>
> Many think that the skin of the blister acts as a dressing and prevents contamination of the wound. However, the skin of the blister is not normal and, therefore, cannot serve as a protective barrier. Additionally, maintaining the blister intact prevents application of topical antibiotics directly on the injury.
>
> In the prehospital setting, blisters are generally best left alone during the relatively short transport time—in most cases, to the hospital where the burn injury can be managed in a cleaner environment. Blisters that have already ruptured should be covered with a clean, dry dressing.

Superficial dermal burns go into the papillary dermis. These wounds blanch with pressure and the blood flow to the dermis increases over that of normal skin because of vasodilation. These wounds are painful. A deep partial-thickness burn involves destruction of most of the dermal layer, with few viable epidermal cells. Blisters do not generally form because the non-viable tissue is thick and adheres to underlying viable dermis (eschar). This compromises blood flow, and it is often difficult to distinguish between a deep partial-thickness and a full-thickness burn.

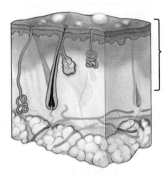

Figure 8-2 Partial thickness burn.
© National Association of Emergency Medical Technicians.

Partial thickness
(second degree)

• Blistering
• Painful
• Glistening wound bed

QUICK TIP

The presence of sensation to touch indicates that the burn is a deep partial-thickness injury.

Full-Thickness Burns

A full-thickness burn results in complete destruction of the epidermis and dermis, leaving nothing to repopulate the wound.

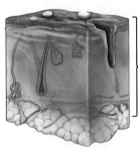

Figure 8-3 Full-thickness burn.
© National Association of Emergency Medical Technicians.

Full thickness
(third degree)

• Leathery
• White to charred
• Dead tissue
• Victims will have pain from burned areas adjacent to the full-thickness burn.

Full-thickness burns can have several appearances. Most appear as thick, dry, white, leathery burns, regardless of the patient's race or skin color. This thick, leathery damaged skin is referred to as eschar.

Full-Thickness Burns Are a Pain

There is a common misconception that full-thickness burns are pain free because the injury destroys the nerve endings in the burned tissue. Patients with these burns have varying degrees of pain. Full-thickness burns are typically surrounded by areas of partial- and superficial-thickness burns. The nerves in these areas are intact and continue to transmit pain sensation.

Subdermal Burns

Subdermal burns not only burn all the layers of the skin but also burn underlying fat, muscles, bone, or internal organs. These burns are full-thickness burns with deep tissue damage.

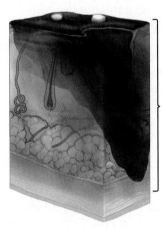

Fourth degree
(full thickness with
deep tissue damage)

Figure 8-4 Example of subdermal burn with charring of the skin and visible thrombosis of blood vessels.
© National Association of Emergency Medical Technicians.

FOR MORE INFORMATION

Refer to the "Burn Characteristics" section of Chapter 13: Burn Injuries.

Assessment of the Burn Patient

Aside from burn-related compromise of the airway or breathing, burns by themselves are not typically an immediately life-threatening injury. The overall appearance of the burn can be dramatic, so be mindful that the patient may also have suffered from a mechanical trauma and may have less apparent, internal injuries that pose a more immediate life threat.

Control of Severe External Bleeding

Burn patients are trauma patients, and they may have injuries other than the obvious burn injuries. It is vital to assess for other, less obvious internal injuries that may be more immediately life threatening. For example, in an attempt to escape being burned, a patient may leap from the window of a building; elements of the burning structure may collapse and fall on the patient; or the patient may be trapped in the burning wreckage of a motor vehicle crash.

Airway

Burn injury is a subset of acute traumatic injury, so as in all trauma patients, you need to pay attention to the airway. Thermal injury from acute exposure to flame can cause swelling of the airway above the level of the vocal cords and can occlude the airway. If you are likely to have a long transport time, you need to be particularly vigilant about airway assessment. Airway management in the burn patient is more challenging when there is smoke injury, or when the initial thermal injury is from fire in an enclosed space. Direct thermal insult to the upper airways results in edema, leading to progressive swelling of mucosa, which can increase resistance to the inflow of air during inhalation. Initially, you should give 100% humidified oxygen to all patients when no signs of obvious respiratory distress are present. The patient should be thoroughly inspected, paying particular attention to the presence of signs of airway burns, such as burns around the mouth and nares, burned mucosa, and burned nares. Also look for chest rise and circumferential torso burns, which may restrict adequate chest rise and ventilation.

Breathing

In the event of a circumferential chest wall burn, the chest wall compliance decreases to such an extent that it interferes with the patient's ability to inhale. In such cases, the receiving facility may need to perform an escharotomy to relieve this tension. Deep airway burns can result in pulmonary damage.

Circulation

The process of evaluating and managing circulation includes:

- The measurement of blood pressure
- Evaluation of circumferential burns
- Establishment of intravenous (IV) access

Obtaining an accurate measurement of blood pressure becomes difficult or impossible with burns to the extremities; if a blood pressure can be obtained, it may not correctly reflect systemic arterial blood pressure because of full-thickness burns and edema of the extremities.

> QUICK TIP
>
> Even if the patient has adequate arterial blood pressure, distal limb perfusion may be critically reduced because of circumferential injuries. Evaluate burned extremities elevated during transport to reduce the degree of swelling in the affected limb.

You need to establish IV access with two large-bore IV catheters capable of the rapid flow rate needed for large-volume resuscitation for burns that involve more than 20% of the TBSA. Ideally, the IV catheters should not be placed through or next to burned tissue; however, placement through the burn is appropriate if there are no alternative sites available. Do not forget to start IO access if IV access proves to be too difficult.

Disability

A source of life-threatening neurologic disability unique to burn victims is the effect of inhaled toxins such as carbon monoxide and hydrogen cyanide gas. These toxins can lead to asphyxiation.

Expose/Environment

The next priority is to expose the patient completely to assess the patient's entire body. In addition, controlling the environmental temperature is critical when caring for patients with large burns. Patients with large surface area burns cannot retain their own body heat and are susceptible to hypothermia. The burn leads to vasodilation in the skin, which allows for increased heat loss. In addition, as open burn wounds weep and leak fluid, evaporation hastens the body's heat loss.

> QUICK TIP
>
> Make every effort to preserve the patient's body temperature.

PROGRESSIVE CASE STUDY 1: PART 2

You assess the child's vital signs as part of the secondary survey and find the following:

- Blood pressure: 64/32 mm Hg
- Heart rate and quality: 132 beats/min, with weak brachial pulses
- Ventilation rate: 32 breaths/min
- SpO$_2$: 98%/O$_2$
- End-tidal carbon dioxide (ETCO$_2$): 40 mm Hg
- Skin condition and temperature: cool, pale, and dry
- Temperature: 95.6°F (35°C)
- Pain: cries in pain 10/10
- Pediatric GCS score: 15 (E4, V5, M6)

Questions:

- Is advanced airway management indicated for this patient?
- What physical assessment finding indicates the potential for respiratory compromise?
- Based on what we know about the patient, what are our management options?
- What percentage of body area has been burned?
- What assessment methods are available to evaluate burn size in the prehospital setting?
- What are the initial actions you should take when managing a burn injury?
- How should you manage blisters from burn injuries?
- What tool would you use to guide fluid resuscitation of a burn patient? Is fluid resuscitation indicated in this child? Why?
- How is fluid resuscitation modified for pediatric patients?
- What is the rule of ten for burn resuscitation?

Burn Size Estimation (Assessment)

Once the primary and secondary surveys are complete, you can assess the burn. Burn patients lose fluids, and this causes blood to get thicker and thicker, making circulation more and more difficult. This form of shock takes hours to develop. A burn patient who is in shock at the accident scene is probably losing blood from an associated injury. Fluid resuscitation in the burn patient is important because you need to resuscitate the patient appropriately and prevent complications associated with hypovolemic shock from burn injury. Burn size determination can also be used as a tool for stratifying injury severity and triage. The most widely applied method is the rule of nines, which applies the principle that major regions of the body in adults are considered to be 9% of the TBSA. The perineum, or genital area, represents 1%. The palm of the patient's hand (with the fingers) is a good estimate of 1% body surface area (BSA).

Dressings

Before transport, you need to dress the wounds. The goal of the dressings is to prevent ongoing contamination and prevent airflow over the wounds, which will help with pain control.

Dressings in the form of a dry sterile sheet or towel are sufficient before transporting the patient. Several layers of blankets are then placed over the sterile burn sheets to help the patient maintain body heat. Topical antibiotic ointments and creams should not be applied until the patient has been evaluated by the burn center.

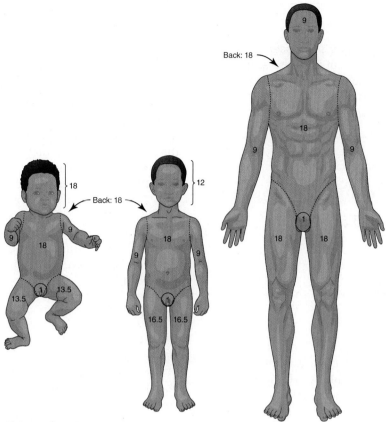

Figure 8-5 Rule of nines.
© Jones & Bartlett Learning.

Age Matters

Estimation of burn size in children is different than in adults due to the increase of TBSA in the head. Additionally, the proportion of TBSA of children's heads and lower extremities differs with age in children. The Lund-Browder chart considers age-related changes in children. Using these charts, you can map the burn and then determine burn size based on an accompanying reference table. This method requires drawing a map of the burns and then converting the map to a calculated burned surface area. The complexity of this method makes it difficult to use in a prehospital situation.

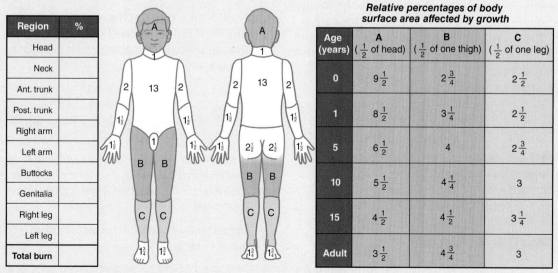

Region	%
Head	
Neck	
Ant. trunk	
Post. trunk	
Right arm	
Left arm	
Buttocks	
Genitalia	
Right leg	
Left leg	
Total burn	

Relative percentages of body surface area affected by growth

Age (years)	A ($\frac{1}{2}$ of head)	B ($\frac{1}{2}$ of one thigh)	C ($\frac{1}{2}$ of one leg)
0	$9\frac{1}{2}$	$2\frac{3}{4}$	$2\frac{1}{2}$
1	$8\frac{1}{2}$	$3\frac{1}{4}$	$2\frac{1}{2}$
5	$6\frac{1}{2}$	4	$2\frac{3}{4}$
10	$5\frac{1}{2}$	$4\frac{1}{4}$	3
15	$4\frac{1}{2}$	$4\frac{1}{2}$	$3\frac{1}{4}$
Adult	$3\frac{1}{2}$	$4\frac{3}{4}$	3

Figure 8-6 Lund-Browder chart.
Modified from Lund, C. C., and Browder, N. C. *Surg. Gynecol. Obstet*. 1944; 79:352-358.

FOR MORE INFORMATION

Refer to the "Burn Assessment" section of Chapter 13: Burn Injuries.

Management

Initial Burn Care

The first step in the care of a burn patient is to stop the burning process. The most effective way of stopping the burning is irrigation with copious volumes of room temperature water. However, this method of cooling should not be done in patients with more than 10% BSA burns, otherwise you will cool the burns locally but the patient will become hypothermic.

QUICK TIP

The application of ice will stop the burning and provide analgesia, but it will also increase the extent of tissue damage in the zone of stasis. Application of ice or cold water is harmful to the patient.

To effectively dress a recent burn, apply sterile, nonadherent dressings and cover the area with a clean, dry sheet. The dressing will prevent ongoing environmental contamination while helping to prevent the patient from experiencing pain from air flowing over the exposed nerve endings.

QUICK TIP

If a sheet is not readily available, substitute a sterile surgical gown, drapes, towels, or Mylar rescue blanket.

Fluid Replacement

The goal of early initial fluid resuscitation in the burn injury patient is to replace the intravascular volume and support the patient through the hypovolemia in the first 24 to 48 hours. This is necessary in patients with partial- and full-thickness burns of 20% BSA and more.

The resuscitation of a patient with a burn injury is aimed not only at the restoration of the loss of intravascular volume but also at the replacement of intravascular losses at the same rate that those losses occur.

In trauma patients, you are replacing the volume that the patient has already lost from bleeding from an open fracture or viscera. In contrast, with a burn injury, the objective is to calculate and replace the fluids that the patient has already lost as well as replace the volume that you anticipate the patient will lose over the first 24 hours after the burn injury. Early aggressive fluid resuscitation is aimed at preventing progression of patients to hypovolemic shock.

In disaster situations with multiple burn patients, fluids can be given orally in patients with up to 40% BSA burns.

Adult Patient

Using IV fluids, especially lactated Ringer solution, is the best way to initially manage a burn patient. The amount of fluids administered in the first 24 hours after injury is typically 2 to 4 ml/kilogram (kg)/% TBSA burned (using only the total of the partial- and full-thickness burn area). Current recommendations are to initiate fluid resuscitation at 2 ml/kg/% TBSA burned.

There are several formulas that guide fluid resuscitation in the burn patient. The most notable is the Parkland formula, which delivers 4 ml × body weight in kg × percentage of area burned. Half of this fluid needs to be administered within the first 8 hours of injury, and the remaining half of the volume from hours 8 to 24.

Do the Math

Consider a 176-pound (80 kg) man who has sustained full-thickness burns to 30% of his TBSA. The fluid resuscitation volume is calculated as follows:

$$\text{24-hour fluid total} = 4 \text{ ml/kg} \times \text{weight in kg} \times \% \text{ TBSA burned}$$
$$= 4 \text{ ml/kg} \times 80 \text{ kg} \times 30\% \text{ TBSA burned}$$
$$= 9{,}600 \text{ ml}$$

Note that in this formula, the units of kilograms and percent cancel out so that only ml is left, making the calculation 4 ml × 80 × 30 = 9,600 ml.

Once the 24-hour total is calculated, divide that number by 2:

$$\text{Amount of fluid to be given from time of injury to hour 8} = 9{,}600 \text{ ml}/2 = 4{,}800 \text{ ml}$$

To determine the hourly rate for the first 8 hours, divide this total by 8:

Fluid rate for the first 8 hours = 4,800 ml/8 hours = 600 ml/hour

The fluid requirement for the next period (hours 8 to 24) is calculated as follows:

Amount of fluid to be given from hours 8 to 24 = 9,600 ml/2 = 4,800 ml

To determine the hourly rate for the final 16 hours, divide this total by 16:

Fluid rate for final 16 hours = 4,800 ml/16 hours = 300 ml/hour

Pediatric Patient

Resuscitation in burned children is often initiated following a smaller TBSA burned compared to adults. Pediatric patients require larger volumes of IV fluids than adults with similar-sized burns (reported in some cases to range from 5.8 to 6.2 ml/kg/% TBSA burned). Fluid losses are proportionally greater in children because of their small body weight to body surface area ratio. Additionally, children have less metabolic glycogen reserves to maintain adequate blood glucose during burn resuscitation. For these reasons, children weighing less than 44 lb (20 kg) should receive 5% dextrose–containing IV fluids (D_5LR) at a standard maintenance rate in addition to burn resuscitation fluids.

Special Populations

When applying the Parkland formula to pediatric patients:

- The total fluid in the first 24 hours should equal 4 ml × the patient's body weight in kg × percentage of BSA burned.
- Half of this fluid needs to be administered within the first 8 hours of injury, and the remaining half of the volume from hours 8 to 24.
- Pediatric patients (weighing less than 44 lb [20 kg]) receive 5% dextrose in lactated Ringer solution.

Analgesia

Burns require appropriate attention to pain relief beginning in the prehospital setting. Narcotic analgesics such as fentanyl (1 microgram [mcg] per kg body weight) or morphine (0.1 milligram [mg] per kg body weight) in adequate dosages may be required to control pain.

Remember that a quick and efficient way to provide analgesia to a patient with burns is to cover the burns with a dry sterile dressing, as contact with air is extremely painful.

Circumferential Burns

Circumferential burns can produce a life- or limb-threatening condition as a result of the thick, inelastic eschar formed. Circumferential burns of the chest can constrict the chest wall to such a degree that the patient suffocates because he or she cannot inhale. Circumferential burns of the extremities create a tourniquet-like effect that can render an arm or leg pulseless. Therefore, handle all circumferential burns as emergencies and transport patients to a burn center or to the local trauma center, if a burn center is not available.

Is It Child Abuse?

Burn injuries are the third most common injury causing death in children. Approximately 20% of all child abuse is the result of intentional burning. The majority of the children who are intentionally burned are 1 to 2 years of age. Most jurisdictions require health care providers to report cases of suspected child abuse.

PROGRESSIVE CASE STUDY 1: PART 3

Reassessment of the patient reveals:

X: None
A: Patent
B: Place the patient on oxygen via nonrebreathing mask.
C: Start IV or IO access to provide fluid resuscitation.
D: GCS score: 15 (E4,V5, M6)
E: Expose the patient to make sure there are no other burns.

Questions:

- How much fluid should you give this patient?
- For what reasons?
- What are your options for pain management?
- What are the benefits of providing analgesia?
- What is the most appropriate analgesia for this patient?
- What is the most appropriate transport disposition for this patient?

FOR MORE INFORMATION

Refer to the "Management" section of Chapter 13: Burn Injuries.

Pathophysiology in the Pediatric Trauma Patient

Whether or not an injured child recovers is often determined by the quality of care he or she receives in the first moments following an injury. During this critical period, a coordinated, systematic primary survey is the best strategy to prevent overlooking a potentially fatal injury.

As in the adult patient, the three most common causes of immediate death in the child are:

- Hypoxia
- Massive hemorrhage
- Overwhelming central nervous system (CNS) trauma

Expedient triage, stabilizing emergency medical treatment, and transport to the most appropriate center for treatment increase the possibility for a meaningful recovery.

Hypoxia

Confirming that a child has an open and functioning airway does not mean that there is no need for supplemental oxygen and assisted ventilation, especially in the case of CNS injury, hypoventilation, or hypoperfusion. Due to their respiratory muscles and soft thorax, pediatric patients have limited respiratory reserves and can become exhausted very quickly. Well-appearing, injured children can rapidly deteriorate from mild tachypnea to total exhaustion and apnea. Once you have established an airway, carefully evaluate the rate and depth of ventilation to confirm adequate ventilation.

Don't Overdo It

If ventilation is inadequate, providing an excessive concentration of oxygen will not prevent ongoing or worsening hypoxia; positive-pressure ventilations are required.

The effects of even brief hypoxia on a traumatically injured brain can be devastating. A child with a significant alteration in level of consciousness (LOC) can still completely recover if cerebral hypoxia is avoided. Advanced airway management usually is not necessary but, in rare cases when it is needed, it is critical to properly preoxygenate the child before attempting airway insertion.

QUICK TIP

Most of the time, adequate ventilation and oxygenation using good BLS skills, such as bag-mask ventilation, is the best choice for the pediatric patient. Like adults, children die from lack of oxygen in the tissues, not from lack of plastic in the trachea!

Hemorrhage

Most pediatric injuries do not cause immediate exsanguination, but children who sustain injuries resulting in major blood loss often die within minutes of the injury. These fatalities often result from multiple injured internal organs, with at least one significant injury causing acute blood loss.

As in adults, the injured child compensates for bleeding by increasing systemic vascular resistance—at the expense of peripheral perfusion.

Using blood pressure measurements alone is not adequate in identifying the early signs of shock. Although tachycardia may be the result of fear or pain, you should consider it a sign of hemorrhage or hypovolemia until proven otherwise. A narrowing pulse pressure and increasing tachycardia may be the first subtle signs of impending shock. If your blood pressure cuff is not working, search for a radial pulse. A good palpable radial pulse means good peripheral perfusion.

Pay close attention to signs of ineffective organ perfusion, including changes in respiratory efforts, decreased LOC, and diminished skin perfusion (decreased temperature, poor color, and prolonged capillary refilling time). Unlike in the adult, these early signs of bleeding in the child can be subtle and difficult to identify, leading to a delayed recognition of shock. If you miss these early signs, the child could lose enough circulating blood volume that compensatory mechanisms fail.

QUICK TIP

In the child with moderate bleeding, no evidence of end-organ hypoperfusion, and normal vital signs, limit fluid resuscitation to no more than one or two normal saline boluses of 20 ml/kg. The intravascular component of one bolus represents approximately 25% of a child's blood volume.

Avoid over-resuscitation to prevent an iatrogenic cerebral edema. You need to prevent or treat hypotension quickly with fluid resuscitation, because a single episode of hypotension increases mortality by as much as 150%. Careful assessments of the child's vital signs and frequent reevaluation after therapeutic interventions should guide ongoing management decisions.

Central Nervous System Injury

The pathophysiologic changes after CNS trauma begin within minutes. Early and adequate resuscitation is the key to increased survival of children with this type of trauma.

> **FOR MORE INFORMATION**
>
> *Refer to the "Pathophysiology" section of Chapter 14: Pediatric Trauma.*

Assessment

The small and variable sizes of pediatric patients, the smaller caliber and size of the blood vessels and circulating volume, and the unique anatomic characteristics of the airway frequently make the standard procedures used in BLS challenging and technically difficult.

Effective pediatric trauma resuscitation requires the availability of appropriately sized airways, laryngoscope blades, endotracheal (ET) tubes, nasogastric tubes, blood pressure cuffs, oxygen masks, bag-mask devices, and associated equipment.

Stabilization Priorities

The priorities and steps in the assessment and stabilization of the pediatric patient do not differ greatly from that of the adult when the patient is critical. The pediatric patient with a local or limited non-life-threatening injury may allow you to take your time and work from a feet-to-head approach to gain their trust. Outside of that, your approach should still focus on exsanguinating hemorrhage, airway, breathing, circulation, disability, and expose/environment (XABCDE).

Airway

There are several anatomic differences that complicate the care of the injured child's airway. Children have a relatively large occiput and tongue and have an anteriorly positioned airway. Additionally, the smaller the child, the greater the size discrepancy between the cranium and the midface. The large occiput forces passive flexion of the cervical spine. These factors predispose children to a higher risk of anatomic airway obstruction than adults.

Special Populations

Pediatric patients need to have their heads positioned differently than adults to keep the airway from closing. The relatively large tongue in pediatric patients presents an increased risk of obstruction. Intubation may need to be performed with an uncuffed ET tube due to the shape of the trachea, particularly in infants. The shortness of the trachea increases the chance of passing the tube into the right lung.

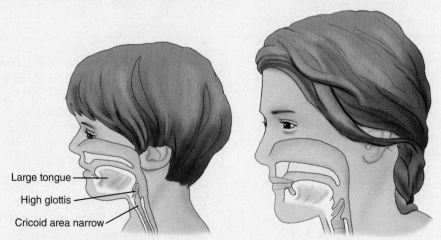

Large tongue
High glottis
Cricoid area narrow

Figure 8-7 Comparison of a child's and adult's airways.
© National Association of Emergency Medical Technicians.

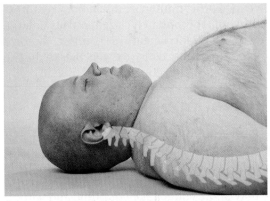

A

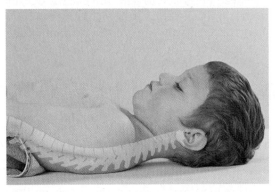

B

Figure 8-8 Compared to an adult **A.** A child has a larger occiput and less shoulder musculature **B.** When placed on a flat surface, these factors result in flexion of the neck.

A: © Jones & Bartlett Learning. Photographed by Darren Stahlman; **B:** © National Association of Emergency Medical Technicians.

Bag-mask ventilation with high-flow (at least 15 liters/min) 100% oxygen is usually the best choice when an injured child requires assisted ventilation. Use a properly fitted oxygen mask and the "squeeze-release-release" timing technique. Watch for rise and fall of the chest, and if ETCO$_2$ monitoring is available, maintain levels between 35 and 45 mm Hg.

In comparison to that of the adult, the child's larynx is smaller and is slightly more anterior and cephalad (forward and toward the head), making it more challenging to see the vocal cords during intubation attempts.

> **QUICK TIP**
>
> Endotracheal intubation, despite being the most reliable means of ventilation in the child with airway compromise, should be reserved for situations in which bag-mask ventilation is ineffective.

Breathing

When hypoxia occurs in the small child, the body compensates by increasing the ventilatory rate (tachypnea) and by an increase in ventilatory effort, including increased thoracic excursion efforts and the use of accessory muscles in the neck and abdomen. This increased metabolic demand can lead to severe fatigue and result in ventilatory failure, because an increasing percentage of the patient's cardiac output gets devoted to maintaining this respiratory effort. Ventilatory distress can quickly go from a compensated ventilatory effort to ventilatory failure, then respiratory arrest, and ultimately, a hypoxic cardiac arrest. Be on the lookout for respiratory pauses, which are ominous signs in children.

> **QUICK TIP**
>
> Central (rather than peripheral) cyanosis is a fairly late and often inconsistent sign of respiratory failure. Do not depend on this finding to identify impending respiratory failure.

Evaluation of the child's ventilatory status with early recognition of distress and providing ventilatory assistance are key in the management of the pediatric trauma patient. The normal ventilatory rate of infants and children younger than age 4 years is typically two to three times that of adults.

> **It Might Not Be a Good Sign**
>
> In the child who initially presents with tachypnea and increased ventilatory effort, do not interpret normalization of the ventilatory rate and apparent lessening of the respiratory effort as a sign of improvement. It may indicate exhaustion or impending respiratory failure. As with any change in the patient's clinical status, frequent reassessment is critical to determine if this is an improvement or deterioration in physiologic status.

With pediatric patients, you will need to monitor pulse oximetry and make every effort to keep oxygen saturation (Spo$_2$) at greater than 94% (at sea level). Because a child's airway is so small, it is prone to obstruction from increased secretions, blood, body fluids, and foreign materials, so early and periodic suctioning may be necessary. In infants, who are obligate nose breathers, suction the nostrils.

Circulation

Assess the child's heart rate and identify whether it is tachycardic, normal, or bradycardic. If the child is bradycardic, go back and reassess the airway. For normal or fast heart rates, look for signs of hypoperfusion (pallor, mottling, poor capillary refilling time).

In a child, signs of significant hypotension develop with the loss of approximately 30% of the circulating

Munchkins Maintain MAP

A child with hemorrhagic injury can maintain adequate circulating volume by increasing peripheral vascular resistance to maintain MAP. Clinical signs include prolonged capillary refilling time, peripheral pallor or mottling, cool peripheral skin temperature, and decreased intensity of the peripheral pulses.

volume. Children will compensate for fluid loss by increasing heart rate, increasing ventilation rate, and shunting blood to the core, resulting in a slower capillary refilling time. Systolic blood pressure can be maintained and then rapidly deteriorate much later than an adult patient. Evolving shock must be of paramount concern in the initial management of an injured child and is a major indication for transport to an appropriate trauma facility for further evaluation and treatment.

A child who is tachycardic with hypotension is experiencing a critical life-threatening emergency (decompensated shock). Stop all external bleeding! Initiate fluid resuscitation as soon as possible, but do not delay transport to a trauma center. You can initiate IV access and fluids en route.

Close monitoring of vital signs is absolutely essential to recognizing the signs of impending shock, enabling you to perform the appropriate interventions to prevent clinical deterioration.

Disability

You should combine the GCS score with a careful examination of the pupils to determine whether they are equal, round, and reactive to light.

QUICK TIP

As in adults, the GCS score provides a more thorough assessment of neurologic status, and it should be calculated for each pediatric trauma patient. The scoring for the verbal section for children younger than 4 years of age must be modified because of developing communication skills in this age group, and the child's behavior should be observed carefully.

Table 8-1 Pediatric Verbal Score

Verbal Response	Verbal Score
Appropriate words or social smile; fixes and follows	5
Crying but consolable	4
Persistently irritable	3
Restless, agitated	2
No response	1

© National Association of Emergency Medical Technicians.

Activity	Score	Infant	Score	Child
Eye opening	4	Open spontaneously	4	Open spontaneously
	3	Open to speech or sound	3	Open to speech
	2	Open to painful stimuli	2	Open to painful stimuli
	1	No response	1	No response
Verbal	5	Coos, babbles	5	Oriented conversation
	4	Irritable cry	4	Confused conversation
	3	Cries to pain	3	Cries / Inappropriate words
	2	Moans to pain	2	Moans / Incomprehensible words/sounds
	1	No response	1	No response
Motor	6	Normal spontaneous movement	6	Obeys verbal commands
	5	Localizes pain	5	Localizes pain
	4	Withdraws to pain	4	Withdraws to pain
	3	Abnormal flexion (decorticate)	3	Abnormal flexion (decorticate)
	2	Abnormal extension (decerebrate)	2	Abnormal extension (decerebrate)
	1	No response (flaccid)	1	No response (flaccid)

Figure 8-9 Pediatric Glasgow Coma Scale.
© Jones & Bartlett Learning.

Repeat the GCS score frequently, and use it to document the progression or improvement of neurologic status during the postinjury period. You can perform a more thorough assessment of motor and sensory function in the secondary survey, if time permits.

FOR MORE INFORMATION

Refer to the "Assessment" section of Chapter 14: Pediatric Trauma.

Management

The keys to pediatric patient survival from a traumatic injury are:

- Rapid cardiopulmonary assessment
- Age-appropriate aggressive management
- Transport to a facility capable of managing pediatric trauma

---

Use the Tape

A color-coded, length-based resuscitation tape was devised to serve as a guide that allows for rapid identification of a patient's height with a correlated estimation of weight, the size of equipment to be used, and appropriate dosages of potential resuscitative drugs. In addition, most prehospital systems have a guideline for selecting appropriate destination facilities for pediatric trauma patients. Be sure to review your protocol prior to arrival at the scene for expedited decisions in critically injured children.

Prehospital Pediatric Intubation: The Great Debate

Data supporting prehospital pediatric ET intubation are limited and ambiguous. In the spontaneously breathing child, endotracheal intubation with or without pharmacologic assistance is not recommended. Emergency medical services (EMS) programs that perform pediatric prehospital intubation should include at least the following.

1. Close medical direction and supervision
2. Training and continuing education, including hands-on operating room experience

---

3. Resources for patient monitoring, drug storage, and ET tube placement confirmation
4. Standardized rapid-sequence intubation (RSI) protocols
5. Availability of an alternate airway such as a supraglottic airway
6. Intensive continuing quality assurance/quality control and performance review program

---

Vascular Access

Fluid replacement in a pediatric patient with severe hypotension or signs of shock must deliver adequate fluid volume to the right atrium to avoid any further reduction in cardiac preload. The best initial sites for IV access are the antecubital fossa (anterior aspect of the forearm at the elbow) and the saphenous vein at the ankle. Access through the external jugular vein is another possibility, but airway management takes priority in such a small space and spinal immobilization makes the neck poorly accessible.

QUICK TIP

In the unstable or potentially unstable pediatric patient, limit attempts at peripheral access to two in 90 seconds. If peripheral access is unsuccessful, try to gain intraosseous (IO) access.

IO infusion can be an excellent alternative method for resuscitative volume replacement in injured children of all ages. This is an effective route for infusion of medications, blood, or high-volume fluid administration.

Fluid Therapy

Normal saline solution (or lactated Ringer solution if normal saline is unavailable) is the initial resuscitation fluid of choice for a hypovolemic pediatric patient.

An initial fluid bolus for a pediatric patient is 20 ml/kg, which is approximately 25% of the normal circulating blood volume of the child. The 20-ml/kg bolus of crystalloid can be repeated once. If a pediatric patient requires further fluid resuscitation after the second 20-ml/kg bolus, the patient should receive a blood transfusion.

You should target a slightly lower than normal blood pressure, or at least a palpable radial pulse.

Transport

Because timely arrival at the most appropriate facility is a key element in the pediatric patient's survival, triage is important in the management of a pediatric patient. Early identification of tachycardia and tachypnea should increase suspicion for multisystem injury and compensated shock state requiring the need for a pediatric trauma center.

Thermal Homeostasis Through the Ages

The ratio between a child's body surface area and body mass is highest at birth and decreases throughout infancy and childhood. Consequently, more surface area exists through which heat can be quickly lost, not only providing additional stress to the child but also altering the child's physiologic responses to metabolic derangements and shock. Profound hypothermia can result in severe coagulopathy and potentially irreversible cardiovascular collapse.

PROGRESSIVE CASE STUDY 1: SUMMARY

You perform a secondary survey during transport and find no additional injuries. The patient is transported by ambulance to a designated burn center. He is discharged to home following several successful skin grafts. The incident was reported to Child Protective Services for follow-up.

Critical Actions:

- Pediatric assessment to identify potential life threats

- Determination of best method to manage this patient

- Reassessment of airway and burns after management is completed

---

FOR MORE INFORMATION

Refer to the "Management" section of Chapter 14: Pediatric Trauma.

Anatomy and Physiology of Aging

The aging process causes changes in physical structure, body composition, and organ function, which can create unique problems during prehospital care. The aging process also influences mortality and morbidity rates.

The process of aging occurs at the cellular level. The period of "old age" is generally characterized by frailty, slower cognitive processes, impairment of psychological functions, diminished energy, the appearance of chronic and degenerative diseases, and a decline in sensory acuity. Functional abilities are reduced, and the well-known external signs and symptoms of older age appear, such as skin wrinkling, changes in hair color and quantity, osteoarthritis, and slowness in reaction time and reflexes. It is important to note, however, that quality of life does not necessarily decrease with the aging process.

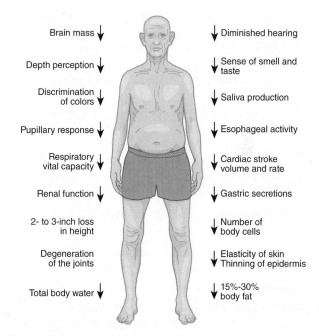

Figure 8-10 Changes caused by aging.

© National Association of Emergency Medical Technicians.

Regardless of whether the patient is pediatric, middle-aged, or geriatric, the priorities, intervention needs, and life-threatening conditions that result from serious trauma are the same. However, because of preexisting physical conditions, older adult patients often die from less severe injuries and die sooner than younger patients. Data show that preexisting conditions impact the mortality of an older trauma patient, and the more conditions a trauma patient has, the higher his or her mortality rate.

Several conditions have been shown to increase mortality because they interfere with the physiologic ability to respond to trauma.

PROGRESSIVE CASE STUDY 2: PART 1

Your unit is dispatched for an 83-year-old male involved in a single-vehicle collision with a telephone pole. Law enforcement is on the scene speaking with the patient who complains of feeling "weak." You notice that there are no skid marks on the roadway. The front end of the vehicle is damaged, and there is no intrusion into the passenger compartment.

Your primary survey reveals the following:

X: No exsanguinating hemorrhage noted
A: The airway is patent
B: Ventilation rate of 24 breaths/min; clear breath sounds bilaterally
C: Radial pulse present with normal rate; skin cool, pale, and dry
D: GCS score of 15; pupils equal, round, and reactive
E: No injuries noted; no significant environmental factors

Questions:

- Why might this patient be at an increased risk for sustaining trauma?
- What preexisting conditions affect geriatric trauma patients?
- What anatomic and physiologic changes associated with aging affect the airway in trauma patients?
- What anatomic and physiologic changes associated with aging affect the respiratory system in trauma patients?
- What anatomic and physiologic changes associated with aging affect the cardiovascular system in trauma patients?
- What anatomic and physiologic changes associated with aging affect the nervous system in trauma patients?
- Does this impact the ability of the geriatric patient to sense pain?
- Based on what we know about the patient, what are our management options?

Ears, Nose, and Throat

Tooth decay, gum disease, and dental trauma result in the need for various prostheses. The brittle nature of capped teeth, dentures, and fixed or removable bridges pose a special problem; these foreign bodies can be easily broken and aspirated and can subsequently obstruct the airway.

Changes in the contours of the face result from resorption of the mandible, in part because of the absence of teeth (edentulism). This resorption causes a characteristic infolding and shrinking mouth and can adversely affect the ability to create a seal with a bag-mask device or to sufficiently visualize the airway during endotracheal intubation.

The nasopharyngeal tissues become increasingly fragile with age. In addition to the risk this change poses during the initial trauma, interventions like inserting nasopharyngeal airways might lead to profuse bleeding even if performed carefully.

Respiratory System

Ventilatory function declines in the older person partly from decreased chest wall elasticity and partly from stiffening of the airway. The decreased elasticity in the chest wall reduces expansion of the chest wall and decreases tidal volume of ventilations.

Stiffening of the rib cage can cause more reliance on the activity of the diaphragm to achieve negative inspiration pressure. This makes an older person more sensitive to changes in intra-abdominal pressure, so a supine position or a full stomach from a large meal can provoke ventilatory insufficiency.

Injuries to the chest wall can compound underlying respiratory changes in older patients. In fact, older trauma patients with rib fractures have a much higher mortality rate and higher risk of complications such as pneumonia, when compared with younger patients. The combination of underlying lung disease and physiologic changes of aging may predispose older patients to respiratory compromise after trauma.

Older Lungs, More Effort

With declines in the efficiency of the respiratory system, the older person requires more effort to breathe and greater exertion to carry out daily activities.

Cardiovascular System

Age-related decreases in arterial elasticity lead to increased peripheral vascular resistance. The myocardium and blood vessels rely on their elastic, contractile, and stretchable properties to function. With aging, all of these decline, and the cardiovascular system stops moving fluids around the body as efficiently.

As we age, our blood vessels build up with plaque that narrows the available blood flow path.

This narrowing can result in hypertension, a condition that commonly affects adults. This is significant because the baseline blood pressure of the older trauma patient may be higher than in younger patients.

> ## QUICK TIP
>
> A common pitfall in the assessment and management of geriatric trauma patients is failure to recognize a "normal"-appearing blood pressure as a sign of shock.

In the older trauma patient, reduced circulation contributes to cellular hypoxia, resulting in cardiac dysrhythmia, acute heart failure, and sudden death. The body's ability to compensate for blood loss or other causes of shock significantly decreases in an older person because of a diminished inotropic (cardiac contraction) response to catecholamines. In addition, total circulating blood volume decreases so there is less reserve for blood loss from trauma. Cardiac output requires atrial filling to help with cardiac output, which is diminished in hypovolemic states.

The reduced circulation and circulatory-defense responses, coupled with increasing cardiac failure, produce a huge problem in managing shock in the older trauma patient. Fluid resuscitation needs to be carefully monitored because of reduced compliance of the cardiovascular system.

> ## QUICK TIP
>
> Take care when treating hypotension and shock to avoid causing volume overload with aggressive fluid resuscitation.

Nervous System

As people age, brain weight and the number of neurons (nerve cells) decrease. Also, the dural bridging veins stretch out and become susceptible to tearing. This results in a lower frequency of epidural hemorrhage and a higher frequency of subdural hemorrhage. The body compensates for the loss of size with increased cerebrospinal fluid. Although the additional space around the brain can protect it from contusion, it also allows for more brain movement in acceleration/deceleration injuries. The increased space in the cranial vault also allows large volumes of blood to accumulate around the brain in the older patient with minimal or no symptoms.

> ## FOR MORE INFORMATION
>
> *Refer to the "Anatomy and Physiology of Aging" section of Chapter 15: Geriatric Trauma.*

Assessment

Although prehospital assessment of the older patient is based on the same method used for all trauma patients, the process may be different in older patients. As with all trauma patients, however, you need to consider the mechanism of injury (MOI) and have a lower threshold for cervical spine motion restriction concerns.

Airway

After establishing scene safety, controlling any exsanguinating hemorrhage, and considering need for cervical spinal motion restriction, proceed with airway assessment. Changes in mentation may be a result of hypoxia from partial airway occlusion or obstruction, so examine the oral cavity for foreign objects, such as dentures or teeth that have gotten fractured or dislodged. Pay extra attention to the patient's cervical spine, which may be deformed and very vulnerable in older patients.

Breathing

In an older patient, reduced tidal volume capacity and pulmonary function may result in an inadequate minute volume, even at rates of 12 to 20 breaths/minute. Because of these changes, you should immediately assess breath sounds even if the ventilatory rate is normal.

> ## QUICK TIP
>
> Keep in mind, breath sounds may be harder to hear because of smaller tidal volumes.

Circulation

Some findings can only be interpreted properly by knowing the individual patient's pre-event, or baseline, status. Expected ranges of vital signs and other findings usually accepted as normal are not "normal" in every individual. Although the typical ranges are broad enough to include most individual adult differences, an individual of any age may vary beyond these norms; you should expect such variation in older patients.

Medications can contribute to these changes. For example, in the average adult, a systolic blood pressure of 120 mm Hg is considered normal and unimpressive. But in a chronically hypertensive patient who normally has a systolic blood pressure of 150 mm Hg or higher, a pressure of 120 mm Hg should be a concern, because it suggests some mechanism causing hypotension.

Likewise, heart rate is a poor indicator of trauma in older patients because of the effects of medications such as beta blockers and the heart's dampened response to circulating catecholamines (epinephrine).

> **Use All the Information**
>
> Quantitative information or objective signs should not be used in isolation from other findings. Failing to recognize that such a change occurred or that it is a serious finding can lead to a poor outcome for the patient.

Disability

You need to take all findings collectively to maintain an increased level of suspicion for neurologic injury in the older patient. Assess the older patient's orientation to time and place by careful and complete questioning. Wide differences in mentation, memory, and orientation (to the past and present) can exist in older persons. Unless someone on the scene can describe the baseline mental status of the older patient, assume that any deficits indicate an acute neurologic injury, hypoxia, hypotension, or a combination of the three.

> **What's the Baseline?**
>
> Establishing the baseline mental status for the older patient is crucial, and it may involve obtaining information from the patient, family members, and/or caretakers.

Expose/Environment

Older people are more susceptible to ambient environmental changes. Their ability to respond to environmental temperature changes through heat production or dissipation lessens. Thermoregulation may be related to:

- An imbalance of electrolytes
- Lower basal metabolic rate
- Decreased ability to shiver
- Arteriosclerosis
- The effects of drugs or alcohol

Hyperthermia can result from cerebrovascular accidents (strokes) or medications such as diuretics,

antihistamines, and antiparkinsonian drugs. Hypothermia is often associated with decreased metabolism, reduced body fat, less efficient peripheral vasoconstriction, and poor nutrition.

> **FOR MORE INFORMATION**
>
> *Refer to the "Assessment" section of Chapter 15: Geriatric Trauma.*

Management

While the management of the geriatric patient does not differ greatly from the adult patient, keep in mind that treatment may need to be more or less aggressive depending on the particular case.

Airway

The presence of dentures, common among older adults, may affect airway management.

Fragile nasopharyngeal mucosal tissues and the possible use of anticoagulants put the older trauma patient at increased risk of bleeding from placement of a nasopharyngeal airway. This hemorrhage may further compromise the patient's airway and result in aspiration.

Breathing

Older people experience increased stiffness of the chest wall. Reduced chest-wall muscle power and decreased flexibility of the cartilage make the chest cage less flexible. These and other changes are responsible for reductions in lung volumes. The older patient may need ventilatory support by assisted ventilations with a bag-mask device earlier than younger trauma patients. The mechanical force applied to the resuscitation bag may need to be increased to overcome increased chest wall resistance.

> **QUICK TIP**
>
> As indicated by lower lung volumes at baseline, large tidal volumes are often not needed when providing assisted bag-mask ventilations as this may lead to unintended consequences such as pneumothorax.

Circulation

Older people often have poor cardiovascular reserve. Reduced circulating blood volume, possible chronic anemia, and preexisting myocardial and coronary disease leave the patient unable to tolerate even modest amounts of blood loss.

Because of the looseness of skin or use of anticoagulant agents, geriatric patients are prone to larger hematomas and potentially more significant internal hemorrhage. Early control of hemorrhage through direct pressure on open wounds, stabilization or immobilization of fractures, and rapid transport to a trauma center are essential.

Immobilization

A cervical collar applied to an older patient with severe kyphosis should not compress the airway or carotid arteries. Less traditional means of immobilization, such

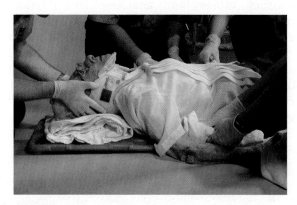

Figure 8-11 Immobilization of a kyphotic patient.
© Jones & Bartlett Learning.

PROGRESSIVE CASE STUDY 2: PART 2

You perform a secondary survey and find no additional injuries. Vital signs include:

- Blood pressure: 60/32 mm Hg
- Heart rate: radial pulses at 68 beats/min
- Ventilation rate: 24 breaths/min, nonlabored
- SpO$_2$: 97%/O$_2$
- ETCO$_2$: 38 mm Hg
- Glucose: 128 mg/dl (7.1 mmol/l)
- Skin condition and temperature: pale, cool, and dry
- Temperature: 97.6°F (36.4°C)
- Pain: 3/10 at throat area

Pertinent history gathering uncovers the following:

- No allergies
- Currently taking 40 mg of labetalol daily
- Past history of hypertension

Question:

- Based on what we know about the patient, what are our management options?

---

as a rolled towel and head block, may be preferable if standard collars cannot be used for the specific patient.

FOR MORE INFORMATION

Refer to the "Management" section of Chapter 15: Geriatric Trauma.

Prolonged Transport

Care for the older trauma patient should follow the general guidelines for prehospital care of any injured patient, but several special circumstances exist in prolonged transport scenarios. For example, geriatric patients with less significant anatomic injuries should be triaged directly to trauma centers.

Treatment of shock over an extended period requires careful reassessment of vital signs during transport. After you control any hemorrhage with local measures, titrate fluid resuscitation to increase intravascular volume status while avoiding potential volume overload in a patient with impaired cardiac function.

Immobilization on a long backboard places the geriatric patient at increased risk for pressure-related skin breakdown over extended transports. Weakened skin structure and impaired vascular supply lead to earlier complications than in younger trauma patients. Prior to a long transport, consider logrolling a patient onto an appropriately padded long backboard or ambulance cot to protect the patient's skin.

Environmental control is essential in geriatric patients with a lengthy transport. Limiting body exposure and controlling the ambient temperature of the vehicle are important to limit hypothermia.

Finally, transport of the geriatric trauma patient from remote regions may be a valid use of aeromedical transport. Transport via helicopter may limit the duration of environmental exposure, reduce the duration of shock, and ensure earlier access to trauma center care, including early surgery and blood transfusion.

Medication Complications in Trauma

Knowledge of a patient's medications can provide key information in determining prehospital care. Preexisting disease in the older trauma patient is a significant finding. The following classes of drugs are of particular interest because they are often used by older people and their potential to impact the physical examination and management of the trauma patient is high:

- Beta blockers (e.g., propranolol, metoprolol) may account for a patient's absolute or relative bradycardia. In this situation, an increasing

166 Prehospital Trauma Life Support Course Manual

tachycardia as a sign of developing shock may not occur. The drug's inhibition of the body's normal sympathetic compensatory mechanisms can mask the true level of the patient's circulatory deterioration. Such patients can rapidly decompensate, seemingly without warning.

- Calcium channel blockers (e.g., diltiazem) may prevent peripheral vasoconstriction and accelerate hypovolemic shock.
- Nonsteroidal anti-inflammatory agents (e.g., ibuprofen) may contribute to platelet dysfunction and increase bleeding.
- Anticoagulants and antiplatelet agents (e.g., clopidogrel, aspirin, warfarin) may increase bleeding and blood loss. Data suggest that use of warfarin increases the risk of adverse outcomes in isolated head injury. Any bleeding from trauma will be brisker and more difficult to control. More importantly, internal bleeding can progress rapidly, leading to shock and death.
- Hypoglycemic agents (e.g., insulin, metformin, rosiglitazone) may be related to the events that caused injury, affect mentation, and may make blood glucose stabilization difficult if their use is unrecognized.
- Over-the-counter medications, including herbal preparations and supplements, are frequently used. Their inclusion in the list of medications is often omitted by patients, who often do not consider over-the-counter supplements as "medicine." You need to specifically question the patient about their use.

PROGRESSIVE CASE STUDY 2: SUMMARY

You complete a secondary survey en route and transport the patient to a designated trauma center. En route, the patient's blood pressure increased to 80/50 mm Hg after 400 ml of normal saline. At the trauma center, the patient is admitted to the intensive care unit for 3 days and is discharged to home following an admission for a mild liver laceration.

Critical Actions:

- Geriatric assessment to identify potential life threats
- Determination of best method to manage this patient
- Reassessment of patient management is completed.

FOR MORE INFORMATION

Refer to the "Prolonged Transport" section of Chapter 15: Geriatric Trauma.

Obstetric Patients

Anatomic and Physiologic Changes

Pregnancy causes both anatomic and physiologic changes to the body's systems. These changes can affect the patterns of injuries seen and make the assessment of an injured pregnant patient especially challenging. You are dealing with two or more patients and must be aware of the changes that have occurred to the woman's anatomy and physiology throughout the pregnancy.

PROGRESSIVE CASE STUDY 3: PART 1

Your unit is dispatched for a 29-year-old pregnant female at 28 weeks' gestation, who lost her balance and fell through a glass coffee table with her arm. The patient is at the front door to meet you. She is attempting to control the bleeding from her arm with a kitchen towel. The patient has significant bleeding from a laceration to her left forearm.

The primary survey reveals:

- **X:** Bleeding from the left forearm partially controlled with a towel
- **A:** Patent
- **B:** Ventilation rate of 28 breaths/min; clear breath sounds bilaterally
- **C:** Pulse rate 114 beats/min; skin warm, pink, and dry
- **D:** GCS score of 15; pupils equal, round, and reactive
- **E:** Laceration of approximately 3 inches (7 cm) to the left forearm; no other injuries noted.

Question

- Does pregnancy cause physiologic changes in obstetric patients predisposing them to trauma?

The woman's heart rate normally increases throughout pregnancy by 15 to 20 beats/min above normal by the third trimester. This makes the interpretation of tachycardia more difficult. Systolic and diastolic blood pressures normally drop 5 to 15 mm Hg during the second trimester but often return to normal at term. By the 10th week of pregnancy, the woman's cardiac output increases by 1 to 1.5 liters/min. By term, the woman's blood volume has increased by about 50%. *Because of these increases in cardiac output and blood volume, the pregnant patient may lose 30% to 35% of her blood volume before signs and symptoms of hypovolemia become apparent.* Hypovolemic shock may induce premature labor in patients in the third trimester.

Some women may have significant hypotension when supine. This supine hypotension of pregnancy typically occurs in the third trimester and is caused by the compression of the vena cava by the enlarged uterus. This dramatically decreases venous return to the heart, and because there is less filling, cardiac output and blood pressure fall.

The following maneuvers may be used to relieve supine hypotension:

1. The woman may be placed on her left side (left lateral decubitus position), or if spinal immobilization is indicated, 4 to 6 inches (10 to 15 centimeters [cm]) of padding should be placed under the right side of the long backboard.
2. If the patient cannot be rotated, her right leg should be elevated to displace the uterus to the left.
3. The uterus may be manually displaced toward the patient's left side.

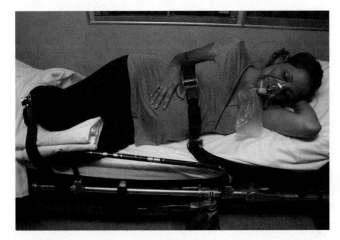

Figure 8-12 Tipping a pregnant female onto her left side helps displace the uterus from the inferior vena cava and improves blood return to the heart, thus restoring blood pressure.

PROGRESSIVE CASE STUDY 3: PART 2

Reassessment of the patient shows:

- **X:** Control bleeding with wound packing
- **A:** Patent
- **B:** 20 breaths/min; clear
- **C:** Rapid pulse
- **D:** GCS score: 15
- **E:** Laceration controlled with wound packing

Questions

- What is special about shock in advanced pregnancy?
- Based on what we know about the patient, what are our management options?
- How would you transport this patient?

Special Considerations

Transport obstetric patients at a 45-degree angle to prevent positional hypotensive syndrome.

Assessment

As with the nonpregnant patient, auscultation of bowel sounds is generally not helpful in the prehospital setting. Similarly, spending valuable minutes searching for fetal heart tones at the scene is not useful; their presence or absence will not alter prehospital management.

PROGRESSIVE CASE STUDY 3: PART 3

Secondary survey is performed, and no additional injuries are noted. The patient's vital signs are:

- Blood pressure: 130/86 mm Hg
- Heart rate and quality: 104 beats/min, with strong brachial pulses
- Ventilation rate: 20 breaths/min, nonlabored
- SpO$_2$: 98%/on room air
- ETCO$_2$: 42 mm Hg
- Glucose: 90 mg/dl (5.0 mmol/l)
- Skin condition and temperature: pink, warm, and dry
- Temperature: 98.6°F (37°C)
- Pain: 7/10 to left arm

The external genitalia should be checked for evidence of vaginal bleeding, and the patient should be asked about the presence of contractions and fetal movement. Contractions may indicate that premature labor has begun, whereas a decrease in fetal movement may be an ominous sign of profound fetal distress.

Management

With an injured pregnant patient, the survival of the fetus is best ensured by focusing on the woman's condition. In essence, for the fetus to survive, usually the woman needs to survive. Priority is given to ensuring an adequate patent airway and supporting respiratory function. Sufficient oxygen should be administered to maintain a pulse oximetry reading of 94% or higher. Ventilations may need to be assisted, especially in the later stages of pregnancy. It is wise to anticipate vomiting and have suction nearby.

The goals of shock management are essentially the same as for any patient and include judicious IV fluid administration, especially if evidence of decompensated shock is present. Any evidence of vaginal bleeding or a rigid, board-like abdomen with external bleeding in the last trimester of pregnancy may indicate abruptio placentae or a ruptured uterus. These conditions threaten not only the life of the fetus, but also that of the woman because exsanguination can occur rapidly. No good data exist to define the best target blood pressure for an injured pregnant patient. However, restoration of normal systolic and mean blood pressures will most likely result in better fetal perfusion, despite the risk of promoting additional internal hemorrhage in the woman.

Transport of the pregnant trauma patient should not be delayed. Every pregnant trauma patient—even those who appear to have only minor injuries—should be rapidly transported to the closest appropriate facility. An ideal facility is a trauma center that has both surgical and obstetric capabilities immediately available. Adequate resuscitation of the woman is the key to survival of the woman and fetus.

PROGRESSIVE CASE STUDY 3: SUMMARY

Secondary survey is completed during transport. The patient is transported by ambulance to a designated trauma center. The patient is discharged to home following closure of the wound and a consult from the OB/GYN.

Critical Actions:

- Obstetric assessment to identify potential life threats

- Determination of best method to manage this patient

- Reassessment of patient management is completed.

LESSON WRAP-UP

- Pediatric and geriatric patients possess unique anatomic and physiologic characteristics.

- Pain management is an important aspect of prehospital care, and you must use good clinical judgment in determining the most appropriate analgesic medication to administer. Do not forget to include BLS pain management interventions.

- Patients with certain types of burns require specialized definitive care offered at a designated burn center.

- Geriatric patients' underlying medical conditions may pose a concern in care rendered.

PROGRESSIVE CASE STUDY RECAP

Case Study 1: Part 1	
How common are burns in pediatric patients?	Following motor vehicle crashes and drowning, burns rate third as a cause of pediatric trauma deaths.
Which types of burns are the most common?	Scald burns are the most common burns seen in the pediatric population age 1 to 5 years.

What would lead you to suspect this was an intentionally caused burn injury?	Child abuse accounts for a large proportion of immersion scald burns. Intentional burn injuries can be distinguished from accidental burns based on the pattern and site of the burn. Nonaccidental burns often have clear-cut edges as found in a stocking or glove distribution, where a child's foot or hand has been held in scalding water. Accidental burns, such as those caused by a child spilling hot liquid, most often occur on the head, trunk, and palmar surface of the hands and feet.
What population of patients is at increased risk for burn injuries?	Older adults and young children are the most susceptible populations to burn injury.
How do we estimate burn depth?	Superficial burns involve only the epidermis and are characterized as red and painful. Partial-thickness burns, once referred to as *second-degree burns*, are those that involve the epidermis and varying portions of the underlying dermis. They can be further classified as either *superficial* or *deep*. Partial-thickness burns will appear as blisters or as burned areas with a glistening or wet-appearing base. Full-thickness burns may have several appearances. Most often these wounds will appear as thick, dry, white, leathery burns, regardless of the patient's race or skin color. Subdermal burns (previously referred to as fourth-degree burns) are those that not only burn all layers of the skin, but also burn underlying fat, muscles, bone, or internal organs.
What are the unique anatomic and physiologic characteristics of this patient that are of concern?	■ Children have a relatively large occiput and tongue and have an anteriorly positioned airway. ■ The smaller the child, the greater the size discrepancy between the cranium and the midface. ■ Therefore, the relatively large occiput forces passive flexion of the cervical spine. ■ These factors predispose children to a higher risk of anatomic airway obstruction than adults. ■ In comparison to that of the adult, the child's larynx is smaller in size and is slightly more anterior and cephalad (forward and toward the head), making it more difficult to visualize the vocal cords during intubation attempts. ■ When hypoxia occurs in the small child, the body compensates by increasing the ventilatory rate (tachypnea) and by a strenuous increase in ventilatory effort, including increased thoracic excursion efforts and the use of accessory muscles in the neck and abdomen. ■ Because of children's high body surface area, they are more prone to developing hypothermia.

Case Study 1: Part 2

Is advanced airway management indicated for this patient?	Yes. Endotracheal intubation should be considered for patients in acute respiratory distress, those with increasing work of breathing, and those who have sustained burns to the face or neck, which may result in edema and airway obstruction. Pediatric intubation should be completed only by experienced EMS practitioners and in situations in which this treatment is without a doubt the best decision for the patient. BLS care has been proven to be equally effective in pediatric patients with head injuries.

(continued)

PROGRESSIVE CASE STUDY RECAP (*CONTINUED*)

What physical assessment finding indicates the potential for respiratory compromise?	In the event of a circumferential chest wall burn, the chest wall compliance decreases to such an extent that it inhibits the patient's ability to inhale. The extremely resilient rib cage of a child often results in less injury to the bony structure of the thorax, but there is still risk for pulmonary injury, such as pulmonary contusion, pneumothorax, or hemothorax. Although rib fractures are rare in childhood, they are associated with a high risk of intrathoracic injury when present.
Based on what we know about the patient, what are our management options?	■ Cover the burn with a dry sterile dressing. ■ Establish an IV for crystalloid fluid replacement. ■ Administer analgesia for pain. ■ Transport to a designated burn center.
What percentage of body area has been burned?	Approximately 1% to 2%, using the rule of palms. In the field, burn size is generally estimated using the rule of nines. The rule of nines is a topographic breakdown of the body in order to estimate the amount of BSA covered by burns. It is important to remember that children have different body proportions than adults; therefore, the percentages must be adjusted accordingly.
What assessment methods are available to evaluate burn size in the prehospital setting?	The most widely applied method is the rule of nines, which applies the principle that major regions of the body in adults are considered to be 9% of the TBSA. The perineum, or genital area, represents 1%. Burns also can be assessed using the rule of palms. The use of the patient's palm has been a widely accepted and long-standing practice for estimating the size of smaller burns. However, there has not been uniform acceptance of what defines a palm and how large it is.
What are the initial actions you should take when managing a burn injury?	■ Stop any ongoing burning. ■ Cover the burn with a dry, sterile nonadherent dressing (sheet). A dry dressing is critical because of the increased risk of hypothermia in pediatric patients. ■ *Do not* use any ointments or other topical antibiotic. ■ Keep the patient warm to prevent hypothermia, particularly in pediatric patients because they are at increased risk of hypothermia.
How should you manage blisters from burn injuries?	In the prehospital setting, blisters are generally best left alone during the relatively short transport time. Blisters that have already ruptured should be covered with a clean, dry dressing.
What tool would you use to guide fluid resuscitation of a burn patient?	Use the Parkland formula. The use of IV fluids, especially lactated Ringer solution, is the best way to initially manage a burn patient. The amount of fluids administered for patients with deep partial- and full-thickness burns involving > 20% BSA should begin with 2 ml of lactated Ringer solution × patients' weight in kg × % TBSA. Fluid is titrated based on adequacy of the urine output. Avoid fluid boluses unless the patient is hypotensive.

How is fluid resuscitation modified for pediatric patients?	Resuscitate pediatric patients using 3 ml/kg/% TBSA.
What is the rule of ten for burn resuscitation?	Researchers from U.S. Army Institute of Surgical Research developed the rule of ten to aid in initial fluid resuscitation. The percentage of BSA burned is calculated and rounded to the nearest 10. The percentage is then multiplied by 10 to get the number of ml per hour of crystalloid. This formula is used for adults weighing 88 to 154 lb (40 to 70 kg). Patients who exceed the weight range, for each 22 lb (10 kg) in body weight over 154 lbs (70 kg), an additional 100 ml per hour is given. Regardless of which method is used to calculate fluid requirements, this is only an estimate of fluid needs, and the actual volume given to patient must be adjusted based upon the clinical response of the patient.

Case Study 1: Part 3

What are your options for pain management?	■ Fentanyl • Adults: 50–100 mcg (1 mcg/kg) intramuscular (IM) or IV/IO slow push to max of 150 mcg. • Pediatric: 1–2 mcg/kg IM, IV, or IO slow push. ■ Ketamine • Analgesic: 0.2–0.5 mg/kg
Would you provide analgesia to this patient?	Initial pain management is accomplished through BLS care, including covering the burned areas with a dry sterile dressing. Burns are extremely painful and require appropriate attention to pain relief beginning in the prehospital setting. Narcotic analgesics such as fentanyl (1 mcg/kg body weight) or morphine (0.1 mg/kg body weight) in adequate dosages will be required to control pain.
What are the benefits of providing analgesia?	Pain management is a fundamental aspect of prehospital patient care.
What is the most appropriate analgesia for this patient?	Opioid analgesics such as morphine or fentanyl are acceptable. Morphine has a longer duration of action, and it may also cause hemodynamic effects.
What is the most appropriate transport disposition for this patient?	A burn center is the best bet. Patients with extensive burns should receive care at centers that have special expertise and resources. Initial transport or early transfer to a burn unit results in a lower mortality rate and fewer complications. A burn unit may treat adults, children, or both.

Case Study 2: Part 1

Why might this patient be at an increased risk for sustaining trauma?	Functional abilities are reduced, including slowness in reaction time and reflexes.

(continued)

PROGRESSIVE CASE STUDY RECAP (*CONTINUED*)

What preexisting conditions affect geriatric trauma patients?	■ Typical findings of serious illness such as fever, pain, or tenderness may take longer to develop in the older patient and can confuse the presenting signs and symptoms.
	■ Older patients may not be properly nourished or hydrated.
	■ In addition, the following might affect each step of the primary survey:
	X—Anti-clotting medications
	A—Curvatures of the spine, such as kyphosis
	B—Impaired mechanical ventilation and diminished surface for gas exchange
	C—Older patients have degeneration of heart muscle cells and fewer pacemaker cells.
	  - Presence of pacemaker and/or defibrillator
	  - Antihypertensive and/or rate control medications
	D—Altered comprehension or neurologic disorders are a significant problem for many older patients.
	E—Older patients have a decrease in skeletal muscle weight, widening and weakening of bones, degeneration of joints, and osteoporosis. Loss of fatty tissue can predispose the older adult to hypothermia.

What anatomic and physiologic changes associated with aging affect the airway in trauma patients?	■ Changes in the contours of the face ■ The nasopharyngeal tissues become increasingly fragile with age. ■ Curvatures of the spine, such as kyphosis, may be present.
What anatomic and physiologic changes associated with aging affect breathing in trauma patients?	Ventilatory function declines in the older person partly from decreased chest wall elasticity and partly from stiffening of the airway. The alveolar surface area in the lungs decreases with age; it is estimated to decrease by 4% for each decade after 30 years of age.
What anatomic and physiologic changes associated aging affect the cardiovascular system in trauma patients?	Age-related decreases in arterial elasticity lead to increased peripheral vascular resistance, and the cardiovascular system becomes less efficient at moving fluids around the body. The cardiac output diminishes by approximately 50% from 20 to 80 years of age. Among patients over 75 years of age, as many as 10% will have some degree of overt heart failure.
What anatomic and physiologic changes associated with aging affect the nervous system in trauma patients?	As individuals age, brain weight and the number of neurons (nerve cells) decrease. The speed with which nerve impulses are conducted along certain nerves also decreases. This results in small effects on behavior and thinking. Reflexes are slower but not to a significant degree. Compensatory functions can be impaired. General information and vocabulary abilities increase or are maintained, whereas skills requiring mental and muscular activity (psychomotor ability) may decline.
Does this impact the ability of the geriatric patient to sense pain?	Because of the aging process and the presence of diseases such as diabetes, older adults may not perceive pain normally, placing them at increased risk of injury from excesses in heat and cold exposure. Living with daily pain can cause an increased tolerance to pain, which may result in a patient's failure to identify areas of injury. When evaluating patients, especially those who usually "hurt all over" or who appear to have a high tolerance to pain, prehospital care providers should locate areas in which the pain has increased or in which the painful area has enlarged. It is also important to note the pain characteristics or exacerbating factors since the trauma occurred.

Case Study 2: Part 2

Based on what we know about the patient, what are our management options?	■ Consider spinal motion restriction, which may require the use of padding in the voids due to curvature of the spine. ■ Perform secondary survey. ■ Administer crystalloid fluids to obtain a systolic blood pressure of 80 mm Hg.

Progressive Case Study 3: Part 1

Does pregnancy cause physiologic changes in obstetric patients predisposing them to trauma?	■ Yes, obstetric patients have hormonal changes that loosen their joints, predisposing them to falls. ■ They also have an altered center of gravity in the advanced stages of pregnancy. ■ They are also relatively anemic, have reduced ventilatory tidal volume, increased risk of aspiration, increased risk of blunt force injuries to abdomen that is already pressurized, and have risk of occult bleeding due to placenta abruption.

Progressive Case Study 3: Part 2

What is special about shock in advanced pregnancy?	Women in advanced pregnancy have an increased blood volume (about 1 liter), so once shock becomes obvious they have already lost a lot of blood.
Based on what we know about the patient, what are our management options?	■ Transport to a hospital for closure of the wound.
How would you transport this patient?	■ Transport this patient at a 45-degree angle to prevent positional hypotensive syndrome.

STUDY QUESTIONS

1. You are responding to a two-car accident on the highway. One of the vehicle's occupants is a 2-year-old boy who was improperly restrained in a booster seat. When you arrive, he is sitting in the booster seat, which is slightly turned at an angle; there is blood on the back of the headrest of the seat in front of him. Despite numerous abrasions and minor bleeding from the head, face, and neck, the child seems calm.
Surveys reveal the following:
   • The child weakly repeats "ma-ma, ma-ma."
   • His pulse rate is 180 beats/minute, with the radial pulses weaker than the carotid.
   • His blood pressure is 50 mm Hg by palpation.
   • His ventilatory rate is 22 breaths/minute, slightly irregular, but without abnormal sounds.
What do these signs indicate?
   A. Multisystem trauma
   B. Traumatic brain injury
   C. Upper extremity fracture
   D. Bowel injury

2. What mnemonic should you use to assess the child's general appearance?
   A. APGAR
   B. CRADLE
   C. RATE
   D. TICLS

3. What are the stabilization priorities for this patient?
   A. Manage exsanguination.
   B. Perform manual cervical spine control, and provide supplemental oxygen with bag-mask device.
   C. Provide pain management.
   D. Obtain intraosseous access.

4. As you continue to assess the patient, you notice that he has stopped saying anything and seems to just stare into space. You also note that his pupils are slightly dilated, and his skin is pale and sweaty. What could be the cause of these changes?
   A. Concussion
   B. Decompensated shock
   C. Hemothorax
   D. Spinal cord injury

5. What should you do?
   A. Administer small doses of mannitol (0.5 to 1 g/kg body weight).
   B. Administer fentanyl for pain.
   C. Give normal saline solution in 20-ml/kg boluses.
   D. Perform mild hyperventilation to lower intracranial pressure.

6. There is a community hospital within 10 minutes of the accident, but it does not have pediatric critical care, neurosurgical, or orthopedic resources. There is a pediatric hospital an hour away. Where is the most appropriate destination for this child?
   A. Transport the child via ground to the community hospital since it is the closest.
   B. Transport the child via ground to the pediatric hospital since they have the resources to treat the patient.
   C. Transport the child via air to the pediatric hospital.
   D. Allow the parent to determine where to transport the child.

ANSWER KEY

Question 1: A
The MOI would indicate multisystem trauma.

Question 2: D
You should use TICLS:
Tone. Moves spontaneously, resists examination, sits or stands (age appropriate)
Interactiveness. Appears alert and engaged with clinician or caregiver, interacts with people and environment, reaches for toys/objects (e.g., penlight)
Consolability. Has differential response to caregiver versus examiner
Look/gaze. Makes eye contact with clinician, tracks visually
Speech/cry. Has strong cry or uses age-appropriate speech

Question 3: B
The survival rate from immediate exsanguinating injury is low in the pediatric population. Since the child is not in danger of exsanguinating hemorrhage, you should provide manual cervical spine control and manage the airway.

Question 4: B
These are signs that the child is rapidly decompensating.

Question 5: C
Delayed fluid resuscitation in pediatric patients has been associated with significantly worse clinical outcomes and an increased mortality rate.

Question 6: C
Because of the nature of the child's injuries, helicopter transport to the closest pediatric trauma center is more appropriate than ground transport to a nearby community hospital.

REFERENCES AND FURTHER READING

National Association of Emergency Medical Technicians. *PHTLS: Prehospital Trauma Life Support*. 9th ed. Burlington, MA: Public Safety Group; 2019.

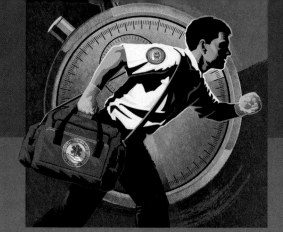

LESSON 9

Summation

LESSON OBJECTIVES
· Discuss the key points in managing a trauma patient—the "Golden Principles."
· Discuss the prehospital care provider's role in reducing the number of deaths and disabilities due to trauma.

Introduction

Medicine has guiding principles. This lesson summarizes the Golden Principles of trauma care. The foundation of the prehospital trauma life support (PHTLS) program is that patient care should be *judgment* driven, not *protocol* driven—hence the Golden Principles that assist prehospital care providers in improving patient outcomes by making rapid assessments, applying key field interventions, and rapidly transporting trauma patients to the closest appropriate facilities.

Principles Versus Preferences

The preferences of how to accomplish the principles depend on several factors:

- The situation at the scene
- The severity of the patient's condition
- Your knowledge base, skills, and experience
- Local protocols
- The equipment available

The Art of the Science of Medicine

Much of the art of prehospital care is based on experience, although there are standards of care that everyone must follow in applying scientific principles to the care of individual patients.

Principles Versus Preferences

Principle—a fundamental scientific or evidence-based tenet for patient improvement or survival
Preference—how the specific prehospital care provider achieves the principle

The preference used to accomplish the principle depends on several factors:

- Situation that exists
- Condition of the patient
- Fund of knowledge, skills, and experience of the prehospital care provider
- Local protocols
- Equipment available

PROGRESSIVE CASE STUDY: PART 1

You respond to a single-vehicle crash into a tree on a rural road in a wooded area. The weather is clear and sunny. There is no other traffic on the road. Upon examining the scene, you notice a bull's-eye fracture of the windshield.

Questions:
- How does this situation affect spinal immobilization?
- How does the situation change if there is gas dripping from the gas tank?

Situation

The situation involves all of the factors at a scene that can affect what care is provided to a patient. These include, but are not limited to:

- Hazards on the scene
- Number of patients involved
- Location of the patient
- Position of the vehicle
- Contamination or hazardous materials concerns
- Fire or potential for fire
- Weather
- Scene control and security by law enforcement
- Time/distance to medical care, including the capabilities of the closest hospital versus the nearest trauma center
- Number of prehospital care providers and other possible helpers on the scene
- Bystanders
- Transportation available on the scene
- Other transportation available at a distance (i.e., helicopters, additional ambulances)

Conditions and circumstances are constantly changing and will affect the way you respond to the needs of the patient.

Condition of the Patient

A major question that will affect decision making is: How sick is the patient? Some information points that facilitate this determination include:

- The age of the patient
- Physiologic factors that affect end-organ perfusion
- The cause of the trauma
- The patient's medical condition prior to the event
- Medication the patient is using, including illicit drug use, and alcohol use

Fund of Knowledge of the Prehospital Care Provider

The fund of knowledge comes from several sources, including initial training, continuing education courses, local protocols, overall experience, and skill set. Your level of knowledge and experience makes a significant impact on the choice of preference. The comfort level of performing a skill depends on the frequency with which it has been performed in the past.

As the provider, you might consider:

- Can the patient maintain his or her own airway? If not, what devices are available, and, of those, which ones do you feel comfortable using?
- When was the last time you performed an intubation?
- How comfortable are you with the laryngoscope?
- How comfortable are you with the anatomy of the oropharynx?
- How many times have you done a cricothyrotomy on a live patient or even an animal training model?

Local Protocols

Local protocols define what a prehospital care practitioner is credentialed to do in the field and under what circumstances. While these protocols should not—and cannot—describe how to care for every patient, they guide the approach to patient care in a systematic way that is consistent with best practices, local resources, and training.

Equipment Available

Your experience does not matter if you do not have the appropriate equipment. For example, blood may be the best resuscitation fluid for trauma victims, but it is not available in the field, so crystalloid may be the best resuscitative fluid because it is available.

PROGRESSIVE CASE STUDY: PART 2

The patient's condition includes:

- The patient is breathing with difficulty at a rate of 30 breaths/min.
- His heart rate is 110 beats/min.
- His blood pressure is 90 mm Hg by palpation.
- Glasgow Coma Scale (GCS) score is 11 (E3, V3, M5).
- He is in his mid-20s.
- He was not wearing a seat belt.
- His position is against the dash, away from the driver-side air bag.
- He has a deformed right leg at mid-thigh and an open left ankle fracture with significant hemorrhage.
- There is approximately 1 liter of blood on the floorboard near the ankle.

You have complete paramedic equipment that was checked at the beginning of the shift. It includes ET tubes, laryngoscopes, tourniquets, and other equipment and supplies as included in the American College of Surgeons/American College of Emergency Physicians (ACS/ACEP) equipment list. All the appropriate medications are stocked, including hemostatic agents.

Question:

- What are your management priorities?

FOR MORE INFORMATION

Refer to the "Principles and Preferences" section of Chapter 2: Golden Principles, Preferences, and Critical Thinking.

The Golden Principles of Prehospital Trauma Care

As a prehospital care practitioner, you need to recognize and prioritize the treatment of patients with multiple injuries, following the Golden Principles of prehospital trauma care.

1. Ensure the Safety of the Prehospital Care Providers and the Patient and Bystanders

Scene safety remains the highest priority when you arrive to any call for medical assistance. You must develop and practice situational awareness of all scene types. This awareness includes not only the safety of the patient but also the safety of all emergency responders and bystanders.

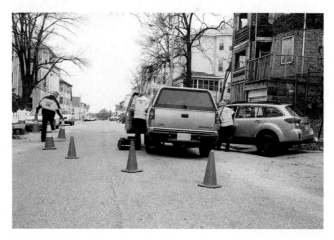

Figure 9-1 Ensure the safety of the prehospital care providers and the patient.
© Jones & Bartlett Learning. Photographed by Darren Stahlman.

2. Assess the Scene Situation to Determine the Need for Additional Resources

During the response to the scene and immediately upon arrival, perform a quick assessment to determine the need for additional or specialized resources. You need to anticipate and request these needs as soon as possible, and a designated communications channel should be secured.

3. Recognize the Physics of Trauma That Produced the Injuries

As you approach the scene and the patient, you should note the physics of trauma of the situation. Knowledge of specific injury patterns aids in predicting injuries and knowing where to examine.

> QUICK TIP
>
> Do not let the consideration of the physics of trauma delay the initiation of patient assessment and care. It should be included in the global scene assessment and in the questions directed to the patient and bystanders.

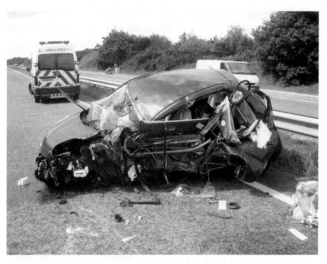

Figure 9-2 Recognize the physics of trauma that caused the injuries.
Courtesy of Dr. Mark Woolcock.

4. Use the Primary Survey to Identify Life-Threatening Conditions

This brief survey allows you to assess vital functions rapidly and identify life-threatening conditions through systematic evaluation of XABCDE (e**X**sanguinating **H**emorrhage, **A**irway, **B**reathing, **C**irculation, **D**isability,

E**xpose/E**nvironment). As you identify life-threatening problems, you initiate care at the earliest possible time, with many aspects of the primary survey performed simultaneously.

> QUICK TIP
>
> Remember that it is a lack of oxygen that will further damage the injured brain, not a lack of plastic in the trachea.

> QUICK TIP
>
> The primary survey is about vital threats. What is critical, and what is not critical? Is rapid transport needed?

> QUICK TIP
>
> With traumatic brain injury (TBI), you must recognize the signs and symptoms through assessment tools such as the GCS score. Focus on maintaining perfusion to avoid secondary brain injury. Maintain end-tidal carbon dioxide ($ETCO_2$) at 30 to 35 mm Hg. Mild hyperventilation is appropriate with brain herniation but must be performed with caution.

5. Provide Appropriate Airway Management While Maintaining Cervical Spine Stabilization as Indicated

After establishing scene safety and controlling massive bleeding, management of the airway is the highest priority in the treatment of critically injured patients. You must be able to perform the "essential skills" of airway management with ease, including:

- Head and neck immobilization
- Manual clearing of the airway
- Manual maneuvers to open the airway (jaw thrust and chin lift)
- Suctioning
- Use of oropharyngeal and nasopharyngeal airways

> **QUICK TIP**
>
> Managing traumatic airways may be problematic. Start with the basics, and know your limitations. Remember, if you don't use your skills, you will lose them!

> **QUICK TIP**
>
> Bleeding must be stopped and perfusion restored! There is no IV fluid better than the patient's blood.

6. Support Ventilation and Deliver Oxygen to Maintain an SpO$_2$ ≥ 94%

Assessment and management of ventilation are other key aspects in the management of the critically injured patient. You must recognize a ventilatory rate that is too slow (bradypnea) or too fast (tachypnea) and assist ventilations with a bag-mask device connected to supplemental oxygen. The aim is SpO$_2$ greater than 94%!

> **QUICK TIP**
>
> Know when to ventilate versus oxygenate! You must be competent with the tools necessary to assess the ventilation and oxygenation status of patients, and you must be able to provide the best method to oxygenate patient.

8. Provide Basic Shock Therapy, Including Appropriately Splinting Musculoskeletal Injuries and Restoring External Hemorrhage and Maintaining Normal Body Temperature

Once you have controlled major external blood loss, you need to consider other causes and complications relating to shock. A fracture, for example, can produce internal bleeding that cannot be observed visually and cannot be stopped through bandaging or pressure; realignment of the fractured limb may be the only means of controlling blood loss in the prehospital setting.

> **QUICK TIP**
>
> Assess the need for volume replacement, which includes the appropriate fluid and volume to maintain perfusion. Optimize oxygenation and temperature control.

7. Control Any Significant External Hemorrhage

In the trauma patient, significant bleeding requires immediate attention. While measures aimed at resuscitation are often the immediate priority in patient care, attempted resuscitation will never be successful in the presence of ongoing external hemorrhage.

> **QUICK TIP**
>
> Life threats need to be managed as soon as discovered. Uncontrolled hemorrhage is a high priority, and a high index of suspicion is necessary at all times.

9. Maintain Manual Spinal Stabilization Until the Patient Is Immobilized

When dealing with a trauma patient, initiate and maintain manual stabilization of the cervical spine until the patient is either (1) immobilized on an appropriate device or (2) deemed not to meet indications for spinal immobilization.

> **QUICK TIP**
>
> Spinal motion restriction should be focused on reducing secondary injury to the spine. Treatment in neurogenic shock should focus on improving neurologic outcome and preventing further damage.

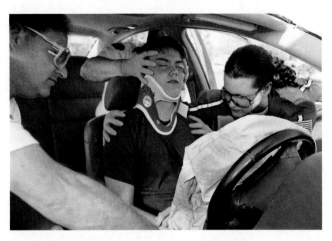

Figure 9-3 Maintain manual spinal stabilization until the patient is immobilized.
Courtesy of Rick Brady.

10. For Critically Injured Trauma Patients, Initiate Transport to the Closest Appropriate Facility as Soon as Possible After EMS Arrival on Scene

Patients who are critically injured should be transported as soon as possible after EMS arrival on scene, ideally within 10 minutes, whenever possible.

Although prehospital care providers have become more proficient at airway management, ventilatory support, and administration of IV fluid therapy, most critically injured trauma patients are in hemorrhagic shock and need two things that cannot be provided in the prehospital setting:

- Blood to carry oxygen
- Plasma to provide internal clotting and control of internal hemorrhage

Keep in mind that the *closest* hospital may not be the *most appropriate* facility for many trauma patients; you must carefully consider the patient's needs and the capabilities of the receiving facility to determine which destination will most promptly manage the patient's condition.

11. Initiate Warmed Intravenous Fluid Replacement En Route to the Receiving Facility

You should never delay transport of a critically injured trauma patient simply to insert IV catheters and administer fluid therapy. No fluid you can give is better than the blood the patient is losing while you mess around with an IV. The priority is to deliver the patient to a facility that can meet his or her needs.

12. Ascertain the Patient's Medical History, and Perform a Secondary Survey When Life-Threatening Problems Have Been Satisfactorily Managed or Have Been Ruled Out

If you find life-threatening conditions during the primary survey, you need to perform key interventions and transport the patient within the Platinum 10 Minutes. If you do not find life-threatening conditions, you can perform a secondary survey. You should also get a SAMPLE history during the secondary survey. Injuries that are not life threatening can make a transfer to a trauma center necessary (think of a knee dislocation with vascular injury).

> **QUICK TIP**
>
> Reassess the patient's airway, ventilatory, and circulatory status along with vital signs frequently because patients who initially present without life-threatening injuries may subsequently develop them.

> **QUICK TIP**
>
> When performing a secondary survey, remember to reassess, reassess, and reassess for life-threat management. Search for underlying injuries if the situation permits, and use the "see, hear, and feel" approach. Obtain vital signs, and treat your patient both subjectively and objectively.

13. Provide Adequate Pain Relief

Patients who have sustained serious injury are typically in significant pain. You should provide analgesics to relieve pain as long as no contraindications exist.

14. Provide Thorough and Accurate Communication Regarding the Patient and the Circumstances of the Injury to the Receiving Facility

Communication about a trauma patient with the receiving hospital involves three components:

- Prearrival warning
- Verbal report upon arrival

- Written documentation of the encounter in the patient care report (PCR)

Care of the trauma patient is a team effort. The response to a critical trauma patient begins with you and continues in the hospital. Delivering information from the prehospital setting to the receiving hospital allows for notification and mobilization of appropriate hospital resources to ensure an optimal reception of the patient.

> **SPECIAL CONSIDERATIONS**
>
> Medications and medical histories provide complications to trauma care. Look for comorbidities in geriatric patients.

> **FOR MORE INFORMATION**
>
> *Refer to the "The Golden Principles of Prehospital Trauma Care" section of Chapter 2: Golden Principles, Preferences, and Critical Thinking.*

Your Role in Reducing Injury and Deaths

Prevention

The ideal is to prevent an injury from occurring in the first place, thus eliminating the need to treat it after it occurs. When injury is prevented, it spares the patient and family from suffering and economic hardship. Emergency medical services (EMS) and EMS practitioners play a crucial role in preventing injury and deaths due to trauma. For example, the World Health Organization (WHO) predicts that road traffic accidents will increase to become the seventh leading cause of death worldwide by 2030 if prevention efforts do not improve. Programs such as "It Can Wait" focus on prevention efforts through public awareness campaigns.

> **FOR MORE INFORMATION**
>
> *Refer to the "Concepts of Injury Prevention" section of Chapter 16: Injury Prevention.*

Continuous Quality Improvement

Continuous quality improvement (CQI) should be an ongoing process in your agency and requires the active involvement of the medical director. The intent of CQI is to improve care. It should never be used for punitive actions against prehospital care providers. CQI is an active process that should include stakeholders from the top down—from executives, to managers, to providers.

Skill Maintenance

Skill performance is a frequently examined aspect of EMS. For example, failed intubations can be disastrous for patient outcomes and may be a trigger for potential litigation. Airway management is critical—failure is not an option!

Remember that prehospital skills are perishable. Regular practice ensures peak performance and maintenance of critical skills. Maintain your knowledge base and apply current local practices.

> **QUICK TIP**
>
> Use a team-based approach with all aspects of training. Integrate basic life support (BLS) and advanced life support (ALS) practitioners for skills practice, and include BLS assist for ALS procedures.

National Association of Emergency Medical Technicians (NAEMT) Continuing Education Programs

As you already know, prehospital care is ever-changing in response to evidence-based medicine. NAEMT continuing education programs emphasize critical-thinking skills to obtain the best outcomes for patients. Current courses include:

- Advanced Medical Life Support (AMLS)
- All Hazards Disaster Response (AHDR)
- Emergency Pediatric Care (EPC)
- Emergency Vehicle Operator Safety (EVOS)
- EMS Safety
- Geriatric Education for Emergency Medical Services (GEMS)
- Principles of Ethics and Personal Leadership (PEPL)
- Psychological Trauma in the EMS Patient (PTEP)
- Tactical Combat Casualty Care (TCCC) for medical military personnel

- Tactical Combat Casualty Care for All Combatants (TCCC-AC) for nonmedical military personnel
- Tactical Emergency Casualty Care (TECC)

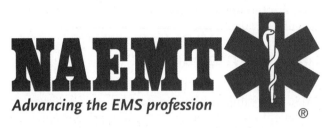

Figure 9-4 NAEMT continuing education programs emphasize critical-thinking skills to obtain the best outcomes for patients.
© National Association of Emergency Medical Technicians.

"We have accepted this responsibility . . . we must give to our patients the very best care that we can."

"What have you done today for the good of mankind?"

Norman E. McSwain, MD

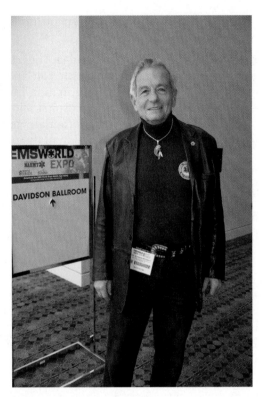

Figure 9-5 Dr. Norman McSwain.
Courtesy Norman McSwain, MD, FACS, NREMT-P.

LESSON WRAP-UP

- Remember, it is often the first decision that determines outcomes.
- If we understand the event, we can aggressively assess for life threats.
- If we address the patient's needs, continuously assess throughout our care, get the patient to the right place in a timely manner, and communicate and document the patient's history, we give our patient the best chance at the best possible outcome.

PROGRESSIVE CASE STUDY RECAP

Part 1

How does this situation affect spinal immobilization?	Some examples of how the situation affects a procedure such as spinal immobilization include:
	▪ Examining the patient in the car; significant back pain and lower extremity weakness are noted.
	▪ Applying a cervical collar
	▪ Securing the patient on a short backboard
	▪ Rotating the patient onto a long backboard and removing him from the car
	▪ Completing the physical assessment
	▪ Transporting the patient to the hospital

How does the situation change if there is gas dripping from the gas tank?	In this case, you would need to:
	▪ Use rapid extrication techniques to move the patient a distance away from the vehicle. ▪ Examine the patient, and determine the need for spinal motion restriction. ▪ Complete the physical assessment. ▪ Transport the patient.

Part 2

What are your management priorities?	▪ You should apply manual pressure to the bleeding ankle to control the hemorrhage. ▪ You should splint the patient's femur and transport him to the nearby trauma center.

STUDY QUESTIONS

1. The situation, the patient's condition, and local protocols are examples of which of the following?
   A. Data analysis
   B. Preferences
   C. Principles
   D. Rapid decision making

2. Which of the following Golden Principles is the highest priority?
   A. Assess the scene to determine the need for additional resources.
   B. Ensure the safety of providers and the patient.
   C. Recognize the physics of trauma.
   D. Use the primary survey to identify life threats.

3. Why should you warm crystalloid IV fluids?
   A. It assists with clotting factors.
   B. Warming increases oxygen delivery capabilities.
   C. It helps prevent hypothermia.
   D. There is no medical advantage to warming IV fluids.

4. What is the Golden Period anyway?
   A. The time it takes for shock to set in
   B. The time it takes to transfer a potentially critical trauma patient from the scene
   C. A crucial period where the cascade of events can worsen the long-term survival and overall outcomes of the patient
   D. When the provider has sufficient time to think through a situation and takes advantage of it through the critical-thinking process

ANSWER KEY

Question 1: B

These are examples of *preferences*—how the specific prehospital care provider achieves the principle.

Question 2: B

Scene safety remains the highest priority on arrival to all calls for medical assistance. Prehospital care providers must develop and practice situational awareness of all scene types.

Question 3: C

Warming IV fluids helps avoid hypothermia. Crystalloids do not transport oxygen and can disrupt clotting.

Question 4: C

The Golden Period is a crucial period where the cascade of events can worsen the long-term survival and overall outcomes of the patient.

REFERENCES AND FURTHER READING

National Association of Emergency Medical Technicians. *PHTLS: Prehospital Trauma Life Support*. 9th ed. Burlington, MA: Public Safety Group; 2019.

Index

Page numbers followed by *f* or *t* indicate material in figures or tables, respectively.

carbon dioxide, and cerebral blood flow, 109–110
carbon monoxide, inhalation of, 45
cardiogenic shock, 73, 76t
cardiovascular system, and aging, 162–163
CDC. *See* Centers for Disease Control and Prevention
cellular respiration, 57
Centers for Disease Control and Prevention (CDC), 22
    Guidelines for Field Triage of Injured Patients, 99, 100
central cyanosis, 158
central nervous system (CNS) injury, in children, 157
cerebral blood flow, 108
    autoregulation of, 108–109
    carbon dioxide and, 109–110
    oxygen and, 109
cerebral concussion, 110–111
cerebral contusions, 113
cerebral perfusion pressure (CPP), 108
cervical spine stabilization, 178–179
chest
    anatomy of, 96f
    decompression of, 62
    visual examination of, 96
child abuse, 155
child safety seats, 8
children
    versus adult airway, 38–40, 39f, 40f
    burn management, 155
    burn size estimation in, 153
    CNS injury in, 157
    hypoxia in, 156
    shock management, 78
    special treatment needs based on physical development at time of injury, 147
circulation
    assessment of burn patient, 151
    life threats management, 19
    in older patients, 163–165
    in pediatric patients, 158–159
    in shock patients, 79
    traumatic brain injury, 119
circumferential burns, 155
class I hemorrhage, 76–77
class II hemorrhage, 77
class III hemorrhage, 77
class IV hemorrhage, 77–78
clavicles (C4–C5 dermatome), 127
clinical herniation syndromes, 116–117, 116f

coagulopathy, 85
colloids, 81
COMBITUBE, 41
communication, about trauma patient, 10, 180–181
complete spinal cord injury, 126
complex airways, 41–42
compression fractures, 129
continuous positive airway pressure (CPAP), 60
continuous quality improvement (CQI), 181
    in intubation, 42–43
cord compression, 130
cord concussion, 129
cord contusion, 129–130
cord laceration, 130
Cowley, R Adams, 9
CPAP. *See* continuous positive airway pressure
CPP. *See* cerebral perfusion pressure
CQI. *See* continuous quality improvement
cribriform plate, 95
cricothyroidotomy, 40, 41
critical thinking components, in emergency medical care, 3, 3f
crystalloids, 81
CSF leakage, 115
Cushing phenomenon, 117
cyanosis, 58, 61

D
DAI. *See* diffuse axonal injury
dead space, 33
decerebrate posturing, 116, 116f
decorticate posturing, 116, 116f
decreased breath sounds, on injured side, 62
definitive care, 98–102
    field triage, 99–100
    transport, 99
        duration, 100–102
delayed injury, 149
dermatomes, 127, 128f
descending spinal tracts, 126
diaphragm, 56
diffuse axonal injury (DAI), 111
direct pressure
    and external hemorrhage, 74
    hemorrhage control by, 16–17
disability
    assessment of burn patient, 151
    life threats management, 19–20
    in older patients, 164
    in pediatric patients, 159–160
    in shock patients, 79–80

spinal trauma, 125–142
traumatic brain injury, 107–121, 119–120
disaster, 21
discoligamentous injury, 129
distended neck veins, 61
distraction-type traumatic spine injury, 129
distributive shock, 73, 76t
diuretics, 78
documentation, in PHTLS, 10
domestic violence. *See* intimate partner violence (IPV)
DOPE mnemonic, 46
dressings, 152–154
    occlusive, 74–75

E
emergency medical care, critical thinking in, 3, 3f
emergency medical services (EMS)
    continuous quality improvement, 181
    practitioners role in preventing injury, due to trauma, 181
    skill maintenance, 181
EMS. *See* emergency medical services
end-tidal carbon dioxide (ETCO$_2$) monitoring. *See* capnography
endotracheal (ET) intubation, 39, 41, 41f, 42, 43, 64, 158
epidural hematoma, 111, 112f
epiglottis, 32f, 33, 39
equipment, availability, 177
ET intubation. *See* endotracheal intubation
event phase, of trauma care, 8
expiration, 56
exposure/environment assessment, 20, 80, 151, 164
external bleeding, control of, 16, 151
external hemorrhage, control of, 73, 74, 179
external respiration, 56
extremities examination, 97

F
fentanyl, 155
Fick principle, 72
Field Triage of Injured Patients, CDC Guidelines for, 99–100, 101f
flail chest, 60
fluid replacement
    in burn injury patients, 154
    in pediatric patients, 160
fluid resuscitation, 81–82, 83f
fluid therapy, 160
full-thickness burns, 150, 150f

ventilation, 36
   capnography, 63–65, 64*f*
   evaluation of, 63–65
   management, in critically injured
      patient, 179
   in shock patient, 78–79
ventilatory devices
   bag-mask device, 63
   positive-pressure ventilators, 63

vertebral column, 126
violence, 22–26
   intimate partner violence, 25
   managing violent scene,
      25–26
vital signs
   determination of, 58
   during secondary survey, 93

W
World Health Organization (WHO), 181

X
XABCDE approach, (primary survey) to
   patient assessment, 5, 14, 15, 35,
   57, 71, 73, 157, 178